CARING FOR JOAN
Insights of a Caregiver with a Spouse Who Has Alzheimer's

by
Thomas J. Rillo

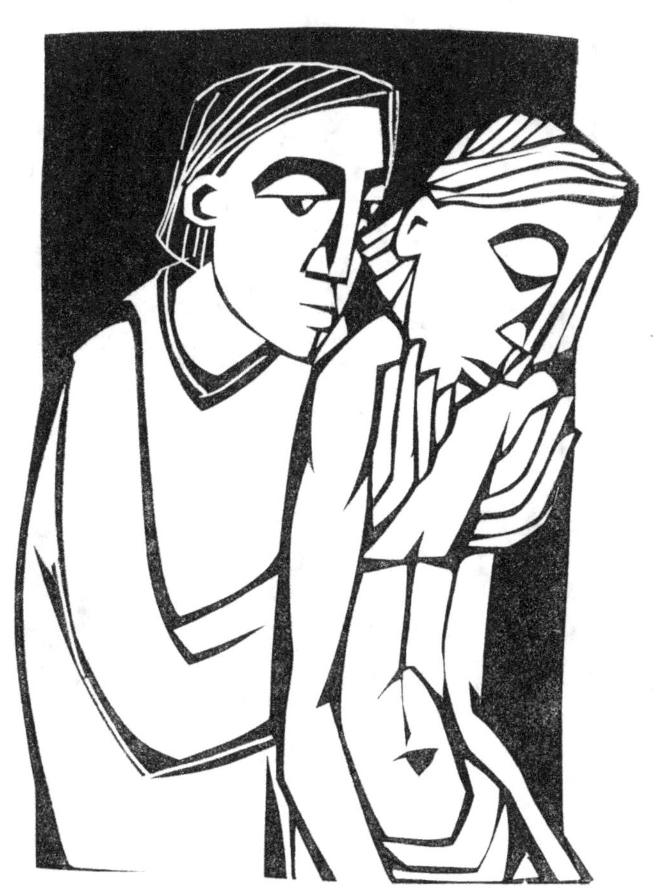

2017

Marriage is a covenant between two individuals. The vows spoken at the marriage ceremony are to be adhered to for a lifetime. The words are sacred and sacramental and should never be broken until death parts the union.

— Thomas J. Rillo

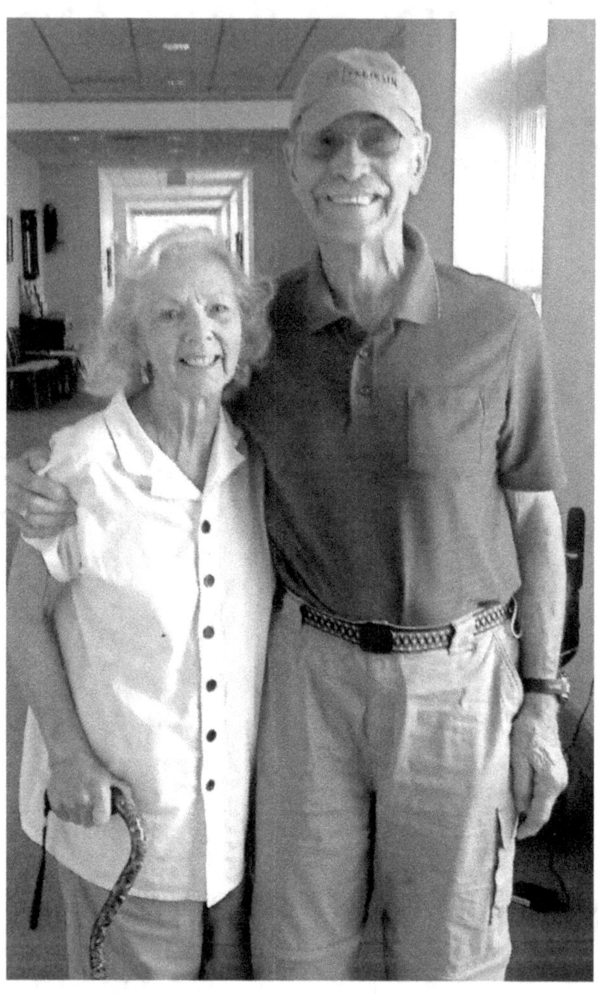

ISBN-10: 1973857286
ISBN-13: 978-1973857280

First published in 2017.
1—2—3—4—5—6—7—8—9—0

ii

Contents

Introduction

Approximately three and one half years ago, Joan my wife of sixty years, began to exhibit early symptoms of Alzheimer's disease (AD). There are listed by various Alzheimer's groups seven stages of AD. Joan displayed stage two symptoms, but I was totally ignorant or could not recognize the symptoms. I was also as a caregiver at the denial level of awareness. As the disease progressed I met new challenges of caregiving every day. It seemed the challenges kept pace with the new challenges of caregiving. I knew I was ill-prepared to be a caregiver for an AD patient. I had four degrees and none of them prepared me for being a 24/7 caregiver. I availed myself of the resources that were available to me. I read a lot about what the experts had to say about AD. In this book, I use the abbreviation of AD to represent Alzheimer's disease. I also refer to Joan and other individuals with Alzheimer's as AD Patients.

I learned that at least 5 million people are living with AD in the United States today. There are 10 million AD caregivers in America today. Joan is one of the 5 million and I am one of the 10 million caregivers in the United States. There are approximately 370,000 new cases of AD diagnosis every year. There are 40 million AD patients globally. This number will double or even triple by the year 2050. The incidence of AD has risen dramatically from 3% affected in the 65-to-74-year-age range all the way up to 47% in the 85-year-age range and older. AD patients live from 5 to 20 years after their diagnosis and loss of the ability to care for themselves as the disease progresses. An estimated 50,000 deaths annually make AD the eighth leading cause of death.

Basically, I focused on the caregiver knowing what AD and dementia are and how to cope with the various stages of AD. I wanted to share what I learned from my experience from homecare to institutional AD care. By no means have I meant to denigrate my wife in any way. This was a beautiful woman inside and out and the outside began to disappear. I kept a journal of Joan's progress through the stages of AD. I have listed the symptoms I have observed in my wife's AD and also my experiences living for part of a day and evening inside an Alzheimer's Care Facility. This disease is not going to go away. Research into slowing the disease has been ill-funded, if at all, in the past. Congressional pressure by advocates of AD research has changed the awareness of support for AD research. For Joan it is much too late for any preventive steps or slowing down of the disease. Well-informed caregivers can do much more in coping with AD in its early stages.

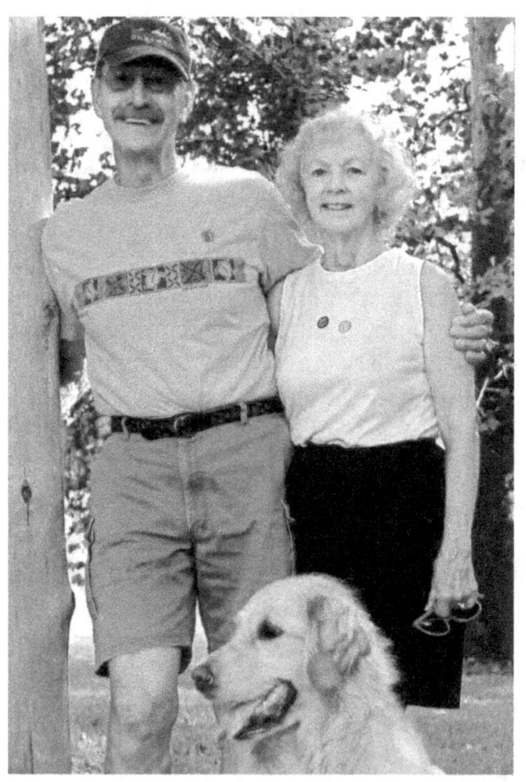

Acknowledgements

There are so many people that have prayed for us during the time Joan has been diagnosed as having Alzheimer's. They are represented by family members, friends, fellow church parishioners, monks of Saint Meinrad Archabbey. One monk, Fr. Meinrad Brune, OSB, has been outstanding in offering prayers both in his celebration of the Holy Mass and in his evening reflection prayers. One family member who was free of job commitments, Dee Rillo, the author's daughter-in-law was magnanimous in her support. She was available and generous with her time. Other family members had commitments to jobs and were supportive of Joan to the point of uncommitted time.

I would like to acknowledge the staff of *Autumn Hills Alzheimer's Care Facility* for their loving care and support of Joan. They are loving, kind, and entirely altruistic in their care of her. This includes the nursing staff as well as the aides. The author left his wife Joan in their care, having the utmost confidence in their unwavering, loving support.

I would also acknowledge Dayna Thompson, MS, LMHC, Alzheimer's Educator, for her counsel and support, especially with reference to the support groups she has organized and urged me to attend. The support group that she recommended was very open and willing to share their experiences as caregivers for individuals with AD and other brain disorders.

I would like also to thank Lauren Hayden, Administrator of *Autumn Hills Alzheimer's Care Facility*, for allowing me to spend many hours per day, not only with Joan, my wife, but also with the resident patients. My observations of these wonderful human beings yielded much information that helped to understand and define AD.

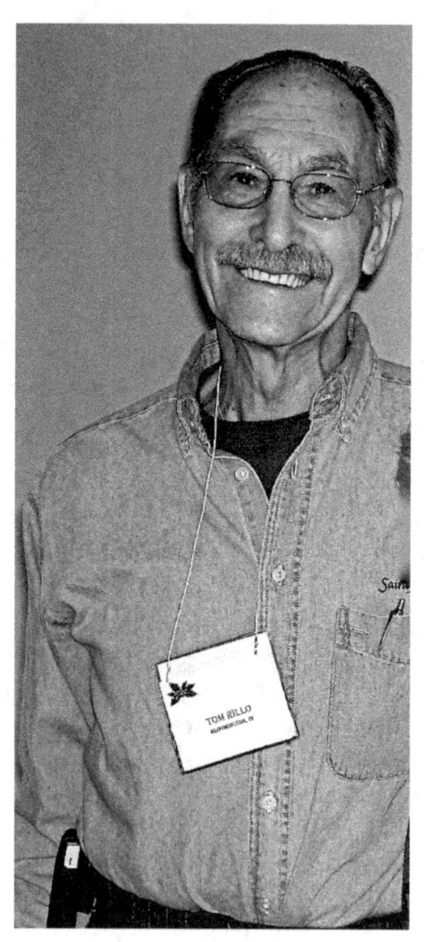

Dedication

I want to first and foremost dedicate this book to my wife Joan. We have been together for over sixty years. During all this time, I never ceased to be amazed at how blessed I have been sharing my life with her. Over the years, she displayed a personality that was replete with outstanding characteristics such as altruism, kindness, compassion, love, a pragmatic sense of the right thing to do. Joan was more than a soulmate. She was my other self. Joan made a home a home with skills highly honed. She was an inspiring role model for our three children and she planned their experiences in activities that were a developmental force in their lives.

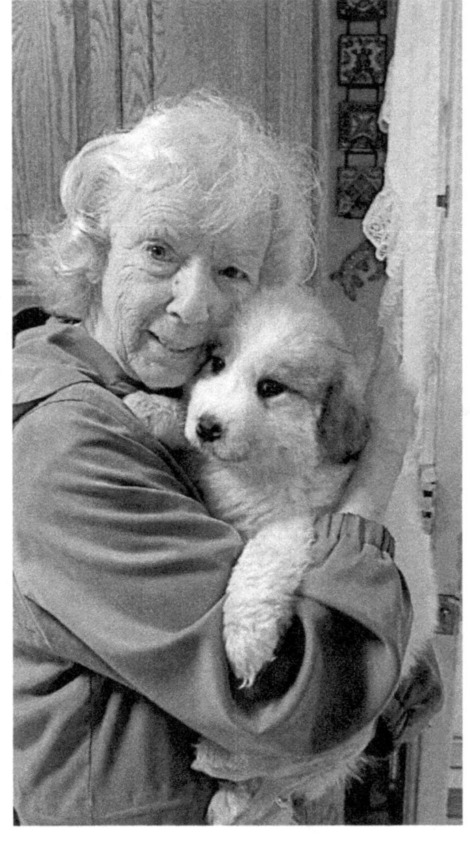

Joan was my rock and my foundation. Without her support, I could never have achieved success, either as a father or university professor. Joan is the subject of this book. In describing her AD it was never written as an undermining of her but rather a chronicle of her courage as she struggled with this monster of a brain disorder. Joan is still Joan alive on the inside.

My secondary dedication is to the ten million caregivers who care for five million AD patients in the United States. Your toil in the AD trenches is exemplary. I am honored to be a member of your legion.

Life is not intended to be simply a round of work, no matter how interesting and important that work may be. A moment's pause to watch the glory of a sunrise or a sunset is soul satisfying, while a bird's song will set the steps to music all day long. — Laura Ingalls Wilder

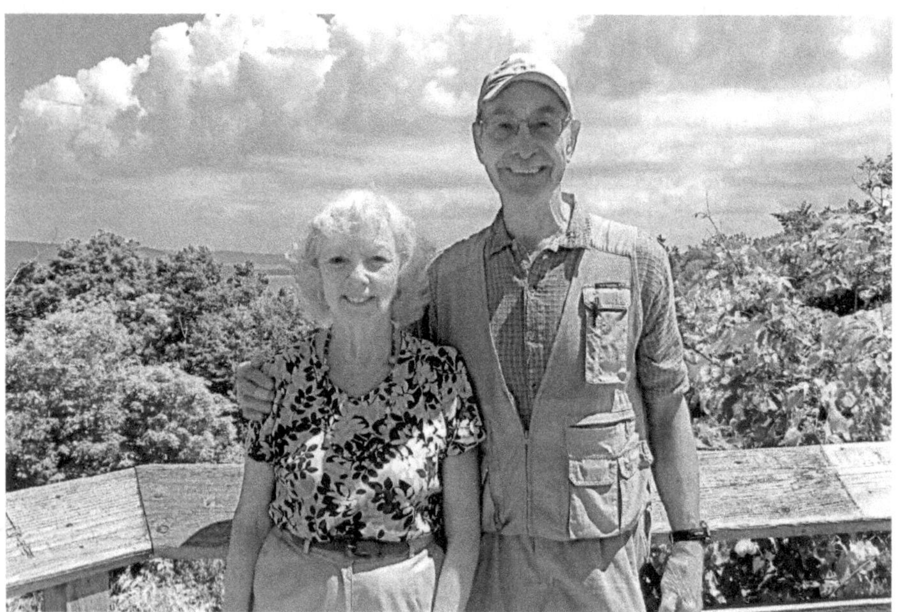

Why I Wrote This Book

It began as early as 2005 when my wife exhibited the symptoms of memory loss. It was just a minimum of forgetfulness and it was Stage one of the seven stages of Alzheimer's disease. There were just simple acts of forgetfulness. Two friends were helping us pack for a move to a downsized home. Nothing to be afraid of and I did not notice any behavioral changes. In 2011 one of the same two friends noticed that Joan was exhibiting symptoms of memory loss. She was forgetting how to get to a location along a route she had traveled for many years. We waited until we could not trust her driving alone any longer. It was hard for Joan to accept not being allowed to drive anymore. It was the last vestige of her independence. This was the beginning of cognitive impairment that was to progress in severity.

As the memory loss continued, dementia manifested itself in Joan's brain. I became a caregiver, and was confronted with many challenges 24/7. Nothing in my background ever prepared me for meeting the challenges that would be confronting me. My four higher education degrees proved to be of no direct help.

I also wrote this book because I wanted to learn more about AD. I thought if I could become more informed about AD my caring for Joan would become much better. I could react to the symptoms with greater clarity and precision. I also wanted to write the book for all the caregivers who might want to read it and profit from my experiences, the good and the bad. I wanted to chronicle the various stages of AD that Joan underwent. I assumed that other AD patients underwent similar progressive symptoms.

Never lose an opportunity of seeing anything that is beautiful: for beauty is God's handwriting — a wayside sacrament. Welcome it in every fair face, in every fair sky, in every fair flower, and thank God for it.
— Ralph Waldo Emerson

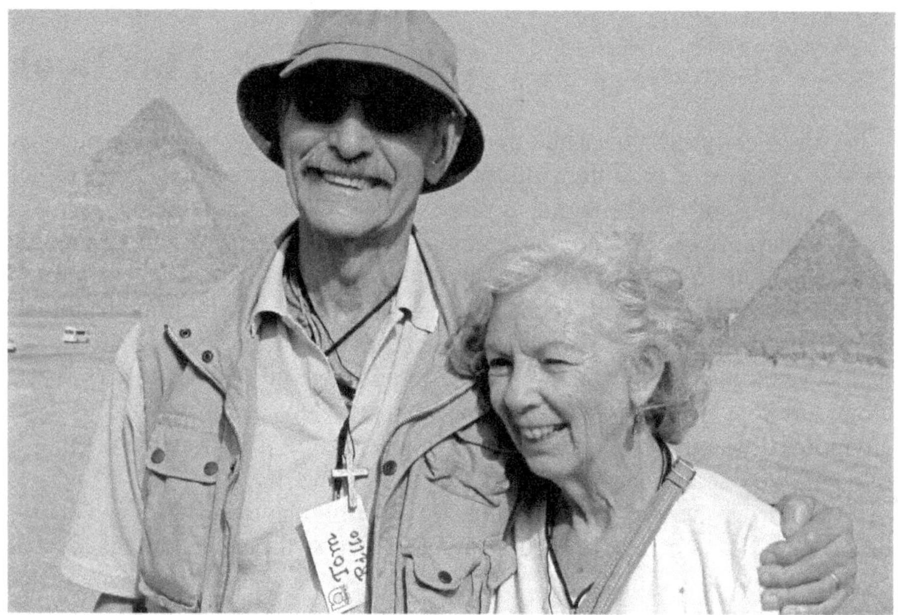

Part One:
How Alzheimer's Changed Our Lives

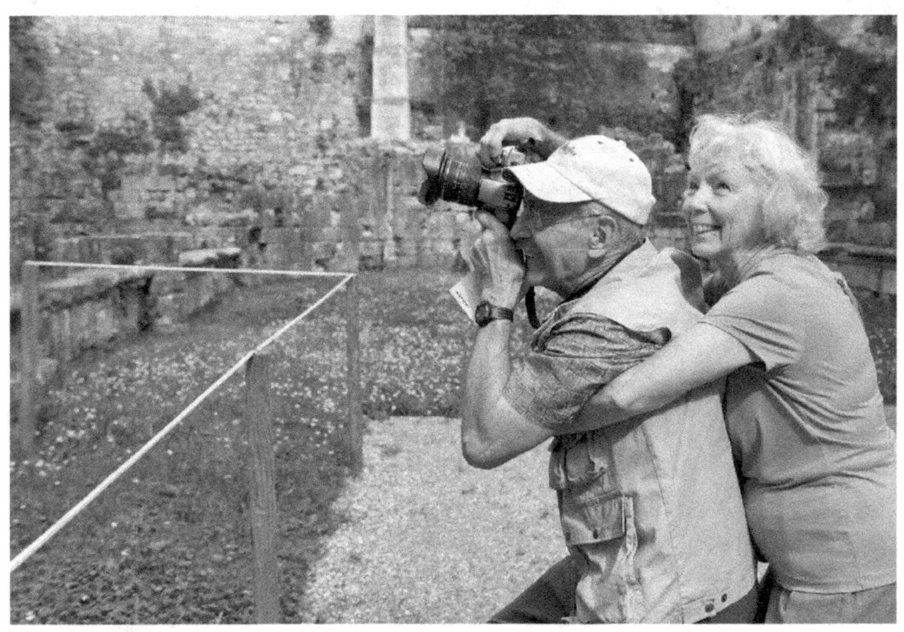

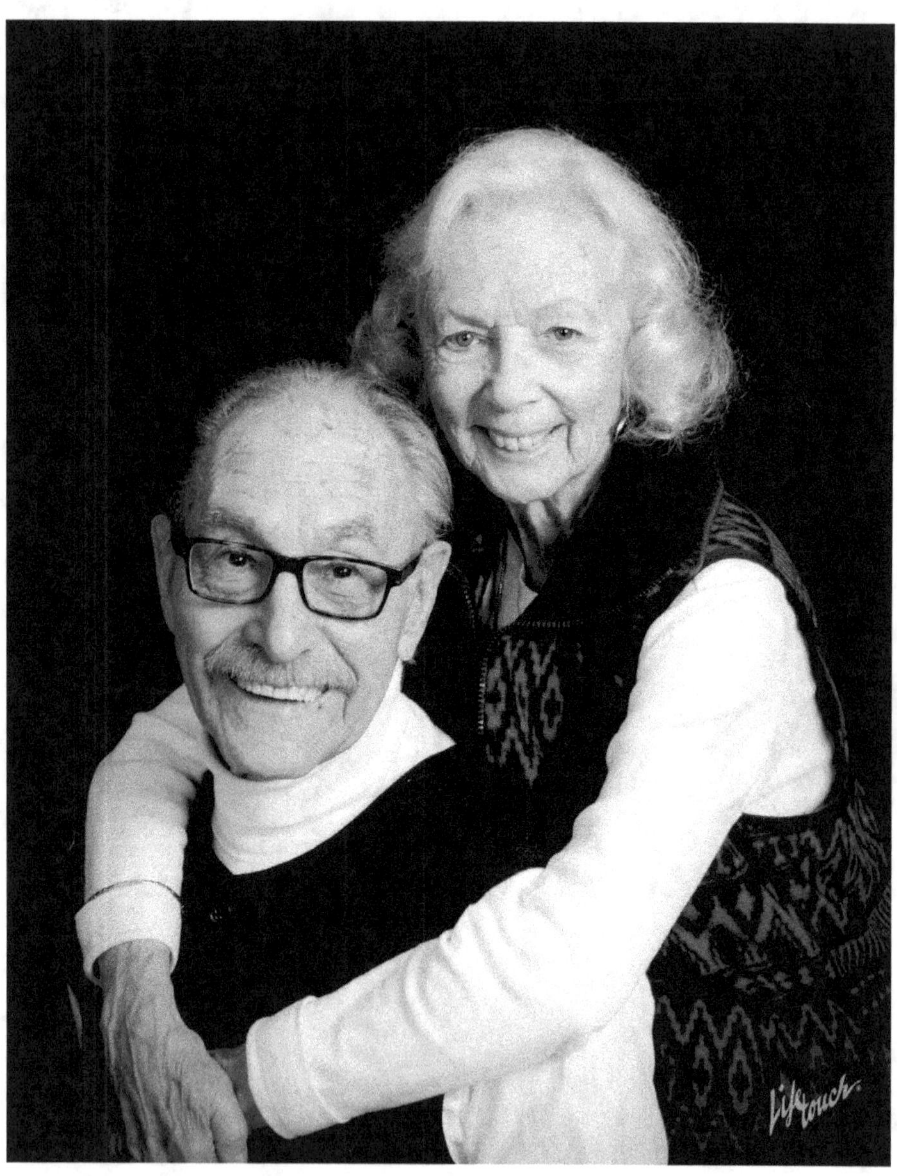

How Alzheimer's Changed Our Lives

Who we were

Joan and I have been married for 60 years.

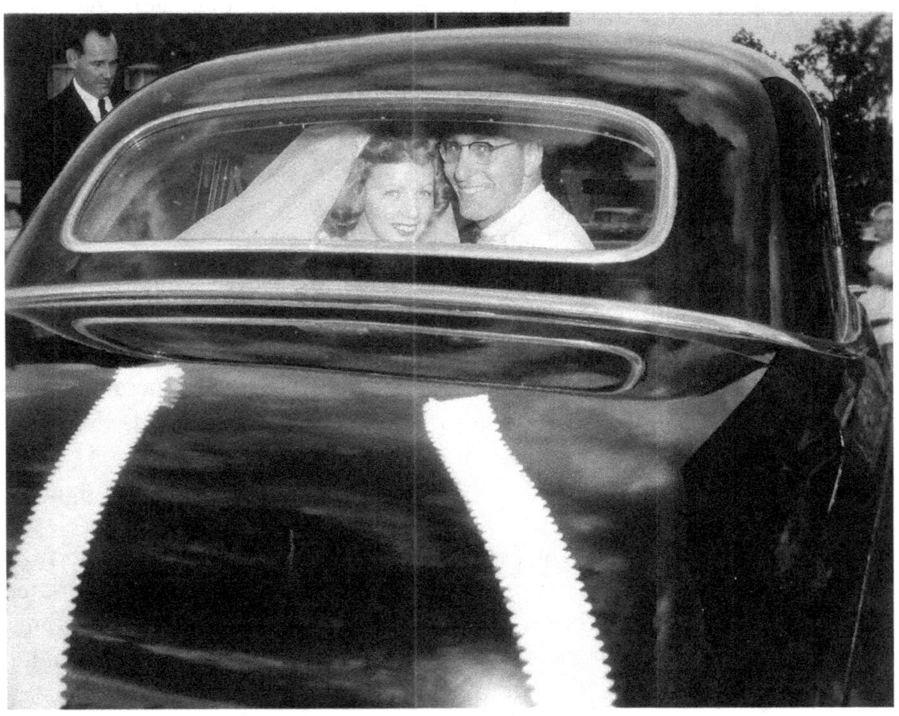

Our marriage vows were sacred to us and I felt that is was a covenant and the vows we said are sacred. I am positive that she felt this way also. We met at the New Jersey State School of Conservation in August of 1955. It was an interesting meeting to be sure. I had just finished my master's degree at Seton Hall University in South Orange New Jersey. The school director at that time invited me to spend a few weeks and volunteer my teaching skills in outdoor education. I had been a staff member at the School previously. He told me to go into the kitchen and get a bit of lunch. I did so and entered the kitchen through a back door and there to my left stood a blonde-headed young lady up on a stool stirring a big pot of tomato sauce with a canoe paddle. I had the audacity to ask her if she was using the proper stroke and the look that she gave would have blistered paint. After my lunch I met with my friend the director who asked me if would take a truck to Indian Ladder Falls located on a mountain in the Pocono range in Pennsylvania.

The director told me that there was a group of ten campers and two counselors camped up there and needed to be evacuated, because a hurricane named Diane was unleashing torrential rains and flooding was expected. I told him that I could not remember how to get there, because it had been so long since I was there. He said: "Take Joan with you for she was there delivering food supplies." I met Joan at the large track-body truck and we proceeded on our way. The rains came just as we were crossing the Delaware River at Dingman's Ferry, PA. It was an old single file bridge with planks for the tires. We proceeded up the mountain and water was running down the mountain road eroding the sides. There was so much water that small logs were floating out of the surrounding woods. I asked Joan if she would put on her poncho and walk in front of the truck until we were free from the floating debris. She did so, guiding for a distance, when I motioned for her to get in the truck. She was soaked, but did not complain. I think at this moment I fell in love with this beautiful girl with such great courage.

I reached the field and fence and faced the truck so that headlights would illuminate my way to the campers. Unfortunately, I had not checked the fuel gauge and we were very low on gas. I got to the campers and wakened them and said: "Just get dressed we are getting out of here." I could hear Indian Ladder Falls was no longer a ladder but a voluminous flow. We got to the truck with me carrying the male counselor on my back for he had dislocated the discs in his back. We came down off the mountain with great care and when we got to Dingman's Ferry the gasoline station was closed because of a power outage. The State troopers allowed me to cross the bridge only if I gunned the truck across. We arrived back at the school, and after warming up with hot chocolate, the campers went to their respective cabins to sleep. The next day was clear and bright as it always is after a hurricane. I found the campers' gear ten feet up in the pine trees. They would have perished, if I hadn't driven up there with Joan to take them to safety. I met

Joan in a hurricane and I like to say that it has been a hurricane ever since. Two years later we were married.

I am seven and a half years older than Joan. Despite this age difference we were very compatible. We were both college graduates. Joan holds a bachelor's degree in education and a master's degrees in biology. I have four degrees. My bachelor's degree is in physical education and kinesiology. I earned two master's degrees: one in personnel and guidance and the other in outdoor education. My doctorate is in Administration with an emphasis on outdoor environmental education.

Joan was an excellent teacher first at the primary school level and then at the secondary school level teaching biology. I spent five years as a coach and physical education teacher at the secondary level. I received an invitation from the President of Montclair State College in New Jersey to teach, coach and coordinate a teacher education program concentrating on outdoor education. This changed for Joan when she started making her own biology and having children. Her talents in teaching made her an excellent mother, giving the kids a myriad of activities that promoted in them the quest for knowledge and an altruism for their friends and adults as well.

My rationale for writing this preamble is to let the reader know who we were and that the insidious disease called Alzheimer's knows no intellectual, economic or social levels. It can descend on anyone as they age. Of course, the disease can affect a broader range of age groups.

On the Road with Joan

Joan and I did a great deal of traveling before and after my retirement from Indiana University. Because of her interest in Native American culture we visited every Indian Reservation and Pueblo in the Southwest. Our early traveling was well before my retirement. Joan had an insatiable appetite for learning and wanted to share this interest with our family. Consequently we traveled with family and for the interest of any one family member. Early in our marriage Joan convinced me that we should purchase a travel trailer. It was a fifteen-foot-long trailer and accommodated all of our family. Over the years we owned and used a variety of travel campers ranging from the travel trailer to a VW bus type camper. Joan was astute enough to know if we had a camper rig we would use it. Joan had a mind that operated unceasingly and always for the enhancement of our family lifestyle.

After the children became adults and were on their own Joan and I began traveling to other countries. We did two or three foreign country trips every year for twenty-two years. We traveled with just two travel groups when we did not travel alone. The first group was a secular one and emanated out of our local bank. The second group was with Saint Meinrad Archabbey.

And we traveled to religious sites such as cathedrals, monasteries, museums and shrines. Travel was in the format of a pilgrimage. We both worked for the oblate program at Saint Meinrad and were friends with the monk who coordinated the pilgrimages. Joan did all of the necessary detail planning for our travel activities. Her mind was sharp and did analytic thinking in a very pragmatic way. All of these travel experiences Joan planned around my retirement years teaching at an environmental school located south of Jackson Hole, Wyoming.

In 1980 I had accepted a summer teaching assignment with *The American Wilderness Leadership School* south of Jackson Hole. It was situated in the Bridger-Teton National Forest and the mountain range surrounding the school is called the Gros Ventres. The school was located at 7,000 feet above sea level. I was one of two lead instructors, and our students were in-service teachers and conservation educators from most of the contiguous states, as well as some foreign countries. It was a beautiful setting to teach in and Joan and I enjoyed our twenty-three summers there. Joan came out regularly once our children were on their own. Joan was a valuable resource because of her computer skills and organizational expertise. She handled every assignment given to her exceptionally well. She assisted me in developing curriculum materials for distribution to the participants in the program. She was great whenever we had serious health issues and especially with individuals that were rescued from dangerous situations. Joan loved riding mountain horses, especially up to the alpine meadows located at 10,000 feet above sea level. Meadows that were covered with bright flowers giving the viewer a tapestry of color.

There were early symptoms of memory loss at the time. We retired from going to the American Wilderness School in 2003, but before that, there were no-visible signs of memory loss. Joan was in the first stage of Alzheimer's that is considered normal for everyone. Forgetting the car keys, not remembering someone's name, not knowing why you went into a room, are all normal behaviors.

Early Symptoms of Alzheimer's Disease

The earliest recognition of Alzheimer's in Joan was by several friends who noticed she was losing some of her memory. It was in 2011 that it became obvious that Joan was having problems. We think that memory is what defines us and gives us continuity. It is a history of who we are. It was difficult for me to accept that this was happening to Joan. When her memory loss reached the stage that it disrupted her daily life, then we realized what was happening. Joan began to have problems completing familiar activities.

An example of this was when Joan sat at a computer while working in the Oblate Office of Saint Meinrad Archabbey. For years she did the computer layout for the quarterly issues of the Oblate Newsletter. She held her hands to her head and turned to Fr. Meinrad Brune, OSB, and said that she could not complete the once familiar task. This was my first serious sign that something was wrong with Joan's physical and cognitive abilities. It both frightened and dismayed me in terms of Joan's lapse into full bore dementia.

Joan began to have problems with spatial relations. She continually asked me the same question over and over. She did not know what day, month, or year it was. These things were revealed during a precursory diagnosis by our primary doctor. She failed to give any answer to his basic questions of time and place. I learned that there are seven stages for Alzheimer's disease. Joan went from stage one (no impairment) to stage two (very mild changes).

An example of a very mild change was when we were downsizing and moving to a smaller one-floor home. A friend came down from the Chicago suburbs to help us with the move. Joan was sitting with the friend and she was observed taking socks out of a drawer and placing them back again two or three times. This was in February, 2005. I learned that the way the disease proceeds and the array of symptoms over time can vary from person to person. It was difficult for me to distinguish between stage three (mild decline) and stage four (moderate decline). The fourth stage (moderate severe decline) was easier.

An example of this was where Joan couldn't find her way to the bathroom, and vice versa, she could not find her way out of the bathroom. Often she had delusional thoughts such as seeing a childhood friend who was in the back yard although that friend lived a thousand miles away and Joan had not seen her at all. That her parents were still alive, though they would be 117 years old today. Having a bowel movement and not knowing that she did it. I know now that the synapse that governs that sensation is now cluttered with amyloids and the glutenates are failing to clear them away. To better understand the various seven stages of Alzheimer's let us examine the symptoms more closely. I preface this by saying that I feel Joan displays some symptoms of stage 7.

Stage 1: No impairments. Only a PET Scan can detect early Alzheimer's symptoms

Stage 2: Doesn't interfere with normal ability to work or live independently

Stage 3: Here we start to notice changes in one's thinking and reasoning
    Forgets something recently read
    Asks the same questions over and over
    Trouble making plans or organizing
    Forgets names or having met new people

Stage 4: The changes that were noticed in stage 3 are now more obvious, and new issues appear
    Forgets details about themselves
    Forgets how to fill out a check with date, amount, or recipient
    Forgets what month or season it is
    Forgets to prepare a meal or follow a restaurant menu

Stage 5: Moderately Severe
    Loses track of time or where they are
    Forgets address, phone numbers, where they went to school
    Forgets what clothes to wear for each of the seasons

Stage 6: As Alzheimer's progresses
    Might remember faces but not names
    Mistakes a person for somebody else; example: thinks her son is her husband
    Thinks parents are still alive
    Delusions that she still lives in her childhood home
    Needs help going to the bathroom
    Likes hearing music and being read to, and looking at old photos
    Difficult to converse with, but connects through the senses

Stage 7: The functions of eating, walking, and sitting up begin to fade
    Difficult to swallow food
    Needs help using knife, fork, and spoon
    Many with Alzheimer's disease stop drinking fluids
    Many can no longer realize they are thirsty
    Disorientation becomes more severe
    Needs help with body needs such as elimination of waste products
    Has to be assisted with brushing teeth
    Bathing is done by someone else
    Their movements need to be monitored; should never be left alone
    Daytime sleeping increases

Joan progressed through these stages, although she did not display all the symptoms listed in each stage description. She showed some of the symptoms in stage 7. This has been difficult for me as a caregiver, especially when she displayed some of the symptoms in stage 7.

For three and a half years I cared for her as she progressed through stage 4. The National Institute on Aging lists three major stages of Alzheimer's. I wish I had known about these stages when I first started to care for Joan. Perhaps I was in denial. That this could not be happening to this very bright woman who was my wife. In the beginning, I was not as well-informed about AD as I am today. I would have known about the challenges I would meet in caring for Joan. Each day brought about new challenges.

If we look at AD in a broader view, we can identify three major stages. First stage is *Mild AD* (sometimes called early stage). The second stage is *Moderate AD* and the third is called *Severe AD* (or late stage). In *Mild AD*, the first stage, people have some memory loss and small changes in personality. Joan did not have a noticeable personality change. She remained the same sweet, kind, and loving person she always was. For me this was deceiving. The signs of dementia were there but I was too uninformed to recognize subtle changes. A PET Scan would have detected a propensity for this monster disease. I blame myself for my ignorance of this disease and the importance of early detection.

Joan's mother exhibited signs of dementia immediately after her husband passed away. She was alone and incontinent with progressive memory loss. Joan transported her by commercial airplane to our home in Bloomington, Indiana. Joan placed her in a nursing home that did not focus on AD care or any level of dementia. She was already in stage seven or severe AD. She died nine months later and Joan transported her body back to New Jersey to be laid to rest beside her deceased husband. The genetic connection was there, but I did not realize it at the time. I only wish there was as much awareness of this horrific disease as there was for the use of tobacco. I feel that if there had been more awareness of this insidious disease I would have dealt better with Joan's early symptoms of AD.

There was a societal denial that AD was a disease and attention should have been directed to the dissemination of information to the general public. The tragedy is that we knew about AD as early as the beginning of the 1900's. In 1904, Dr. Alois Alzheimer was treating and researching a patient with severe memory loss, including dementia. When she died of this memory-loss disease, Dr. Alzheimer examined her brain and found that he had never seen a brain so covered with what he called 'plaque'.

One hundred and fourteen years have passed by and very little if anything at all was done. No research was focused on this disease of the brain. Presently there is research being done, but no cure has been found. The progression of the disease can be slowed down by diet, exercise, and cognitive enhancement activities. The answer to some treatment is in pharmaceutical research, and the discovery of a drug that would significantly slow down the progression of the disease.

With Joan's AD condition, we are well beyond slowing the progression of the disease down. We are long past the preventive stage. Much to my dismay it is too late for Joan. All we can do is make her comfortable and give her love in great amounts. There is an old Amish saying: "Too late smart".

Severe AD is the last stage of Alzheimer's and ends in the death of the person in this stage of progression. In this stage people often need help with their daily needs. They may not be able to walk or sit up without assistance. They may not be able to talk and often cannot recognize family members. They may have trouble speaking, swallowing and refuse to eat. Joan is, as of this writing, refusing to eat more than a little of her food. She recognizes family member faces, but she doesn't remember their visits after they leave.

Life in an Alzheimer's Care Facility

When my wife was first admitted to an Alzheimer's Special Care Facility I had no concept of my spending so much time there. My wife did not acclimatize to being an AD resident. It was also the hardest decision I have ever had to make. I had a feeling of guilt that refused to diminish. So I have at the writing of this article spent 6 to 7 hours daily, 7 days per week at the facility. This equates to 49 hours per week or 196 hours per month. At the end of my sixth month of visitation I will have 1,176 hours visiting my wife Joan. Needless to say that this time has provided me with many insights into Alzheimer's as well as Parkinson's disease, or both AD and Parkinson's.

I have been witness to the progressive nature of this horrible disease. Conversations that I had with some AD patients in six months time were impossible. Processing my words or responding verbally became extremely difficult if any response was there at all. This progressive nature was one of the most significant things I observed. I was able to classify patients by the seven stages of Alzheimer's. Stage one represents normal forgetting and stage two mild memory loss. Stages 3-7 were prevalent among the population of residents. While I was with Joan for half a year in the care facility there were four deaths. Each had the symptoms of the near death. Loss of appetite or not eating or drinking, loss of mobility,

What I learned from my extensive time among AD residents is that they progress toward the end stage at different rates. For some the progression is quick, while others seem to progress more slowly. Each AD resident is different in terms of depression, mood, anger, anxiety, and cognitive impairment. Some respond well to directions, while others cannot process directions. Some tolerate loud voices, while others view it as a threat. Some recognized me each day I arrived, while others processed who I was when they were told.

I also learned a great deal about the staff. The nurses were caring and loving and very competent. The aides were a different proposition. I learned which aides displayed love, compassion and altruism. These aides stood out. Many aides were there at the facility for a short term and did not openly share the attitudes of those who were steady in performance of duties. In our community, there were and perhaps still are over 400 open positions for aides. The pay is very low and not commensurate with the responsibilities entailed in the positions. This is probably true for most health care facilities throughout the nation. It does not alleviate frustration for families who pay the high cost of residential care. Often there is no full measure for dollars spent.

The question lies with the AD patient. Where will this AD patient be most safe and get the best care? Homecare versus institutional care will vary. What is best for the family and the AD patient? The priority is with the AD patient. What can the family afford and are there insurance policies in effect for long-term care?

Joan's Alzheimer's and Depression

Joan's depression began much earlier than her diagnosis of severe memory loss. Her depression moods did not last very long. However, they were intense. In the early stages of dementia, I heard Joan say often that she wished she was dead and could kill herself. By this time, she had stopped reading. Her attempts at letter writing were extremely difficult for her. She would spend weeks trying to write just one letter. She had five or six sheets of paper with only the first paragraph written. Words had lines running through them where she eliminated their use. Joan's handwriting was as beautiful as ever. Her choice of words was sporadic. The recipient of her letter was to be Emily, her childhood friend. It was obvious that Emily had played an important role in Joan's childhood. It tore my heart out just to witness her courageous attempt at correspondence. Beside the date of one of the letter attempts she wrote "I think". This meant she wasn't sure of the date. Again, this was an example of her difficulty with spatial relations. I noticed signs of depression well before Joan's onset of AD. She was showing signs of depression before the symptoms of AD were noticeable.

She often said she wanted to go back to her former childhood home in New Jersey. Joan had no memory of selling the home forty years previously and that it was a floral shop. She was depressed that she would not be able to get to her parents to be with them and care for them. She had done a beautiful job with the funeral arrangements for both of her parents. She had then and even now no memory of the wonderful act of love she displayed in laying her parents to rest. Joan would cry over the fact that she abandoned her parents. She would say the reverse of this when she said her parents abandoned her. This delusional posture came up at least once a day before the early symptoms of AD manifested themselves.

During this time, Joan was making vague complaints about not feeling good, lack of energy, loss of interest in activities that used to give her joy and satisfaction. I was not equipped to deal with Joan's depression. Our primary care doctor was not in favor of anti-depressive drug medications. In his opinion and experience, he felt that drugs were too invasive and would contribute to Joan's memory loss. I noticed increasing apathy, irritability, crying spells, fatigue, problems with eating, feeling of worthlessness and hopelessness, fatigue, and difficulty with concentration.

I was confused about how to cope with Joan's increasing depression and eventually her early symptoms of AD. I could not discover any research on whether depression was a precursor to AD or a risk factor for the advent of AD. However, I continued reading about depression. I think I placed myself at a disadvantage by not seeking professional help to cope with Joan's depression. I was a university professor emeritus with a background in exercise physiology, kinesiology, and applied health. This concentration was at the baccalaureate level. I erroneously thought I was eminently qualified to cope with Joan's depression. After all, exercise was one activity recommended for dealing with depression.

In retrospect, it was a gross mistake on my part. Also, I was in a certain degree of denial because this could not be happening to my beautiful wife of sixty years. She was so intelligent, so analytic and so precise in all that she attempted to do. She had a beautiful mind and I could not embrace the thought that I would be losing such a beautiful mind. I now know that Joan is still Joan within her body and that she is still very much alive within. This is where I hold that marriage is a covenant and that vows we said at the marriage ceremony I hold sacred and will abide by them until death parts us.

I consulted with our primary care doctor to see if medication was an option. He had become increasingly familiar with anti-depressant medications. Even though they were relatively safe and effective in relieving symptoms of depression he was still of the opinion these drugs were not a good option for Joan. He mentioned a drug called Selective Serotonin Reuptake Inhibitors (SSRI's). They increase the level of serotonin in the brain. Our doctor felt that Joan's AD had progressed too far and that SSRI's would have been more effective with Joan if they had been prescribed in the early stages of Joan's AD.

Consultation with depression therapists would not have been an option either, because of Joan's inability to remember what was said or done in a therapy session. In the early stages of Joan's AD, it coexisted for a time with depression and made it difficult to retain any memory of what had ensued during a therapy session. If talk therapy was to be effective in coping with Joan's depression it would have been effective only during the very early stages of Joan's dementia and memory loss. I am told that it might have been effective in the very first stage of AD. Once again I highly recommend early detection. A PET Scan of the brain would be very important for slowing down the progression of AD. It would help the caregivers in their support and understanding of AD. I decided that I would learn more about depression in individuals with AD and particularly depression in caregivers.

What I Learned about Depression

Dementia can cause the same symptoms of depression as AD. When she was in the dementia stage, Joan exhibited the following symptoms. First and foremost was apathy. Other symptoms of depression that I observed in Joan was loss of interest in activities and hobbies. Joan was an excellent seamstress, an accomplished knitter and an avid reader. She also loved to run, jog, and walk. In this depressive state, she did nothing but sit when she was not sleeping. Eventually Joan lost interest in watching television. If the story line was complex, Joan could not follow the sequence and lost interest. Some DVD programs that she liked were *Fawlty Towers*, *Are You Being Served?*, *Keeping Up Appearances* which are all excellent British sitcoms. Any TV program that made her laugh she watched. She liked the *Lawrence Welk Show*, and enjoyed the singing and dancing. Anything too complicated, and I would have to review for her what she just watched.

This was my experience with the effectiveness of music therapy for those with AD. She showed little interest in social interaction, which is another symptom of depression. She was comfortable with isolation and sat in a recliner chair for most of the day. I tried physical therapy exercises with her and she complained that she was too tired to do them. I was an experienced physical therapist myself and had the background and experience in using my knowledge of movement.

Joan had two hip replacements and no doubt any exercise involving the lower extremities could be the reason for her backpain. If I pushed too hard for Joan to do these therapeutic exercises, she would get angry with me. I sometimes took her to the Mall to walk, and Joan window shopped and this motivated her. But her interest eventually waned and we stopped going. I would use a transport chair to diversify her environment, but I was the one who was getting the exercise.

In her depression, Joan would have trouble communicating with me, as she searched for words she could not remember. Concentration became impossible for her. She talked about attempting suicide, especially when she was depressed. Now, in the more advanced stages of AD, she almost never mentions wanting to die. As her thinking process became severely impaired, anger and frustration took over and provided additional fuel to depression. AD and depression have similar symptoms. This was apparent to me. Cognitive impairment is common to both. In both dementia and AD, it was difficult for Joan to articulate her sadness, hopelessness, guilt and other emotions and feelings associated with depression. Depression is much less severe and not as long lasting as it is with AD.

I read that experts estimate that up to 40 percent of people with AD have significant depression. Some of the symptoms that I observed in Joan was some social isolation, loss of appetite that carried over into AD. She became more irritable and easily agitated. On more than one occasion she struck me with her cane when she was angry with me. This I ignored, and it turned out to be the best reaction on my part. Another time she pushed her walker into my legs and swept me off my feet causing me to fall flat on my back. It was in the bathroom, and fortunately I did not put out my arms to break the fall for I could have broken some bones. Joan always complained about being tired and fatigued. I reiterate that physical exercise was always turned down by Joan.

As far as disruption of sleep, this was never a problem for Joan. It is a symptom of depression that never happened with Joan. She sleeps soundly and for very long periods of time. I think that is an escape thing where she is at peace. To the contrary, I was the one who had disrupted sleep. I was constantly on the alert to listen for Joan going to the back room, and many times I would find her in the living room adjusting photos and our assorted collection of figurines, artifacts, wooden bird carvings. Also, her thoughts in her depressive state were characterized by attempted suicide. This concerned me when she walked about the house at night. Like dealing with a sleep walker I kept my voice soft, and used very gentle words in directing her back into bed. Fortunately, these thoughts are sublimated in her present advanced stage of AD.

Depression in the Caregiver

Caring for a person with AD can be emotionally and physically draining. For over three and a half years I was a total caregiver for Joan. I could not leave her alone. We were like Siamese twins attached to each other. I had to take her everywhere I needed to go. All simple errands became very tedious and much slower to accomplish. It became somewhat better when I could leave her with a *Home Instead* person for two-to-three hour periods.

Caregiving became more difficult as Joan's AD began to progress. It took more energy and time as the disease progressed. Every day brought on new challenges in terms of Joan's changing behaviors and loss of her abilities to function alone. I felt at times overwhelmed and wanted to run away from it all.

Fortunately, my spirituality intervened and I prayed a lot. My prayers washed away selfish thinking and negative thoughts. How could I abandon this wonderful person who sacrificed so much for me and for our family?

Joan's AD was in a sense killing physically and emotionally. It was not Joan that was doing it, it was all the challenges and responsibilities that I faced every day. Joan—prior to the onset of AD—would have been chagrined to know she was contributing to my depression. But it was not Joan, but rather a person with AD that was named Joan. Joan was still alive inside and I was watching the outside that was disappearing. Once I accepted this reality, my depression significantly lessened.

It lessened to a greater degree when Joan was admitted to *Autumn Hills Alzheimer's Care Facility*. I now had the mornings free to do the many household tasks and assorted maintenance tasks associated with owning a home.

Exercise both physical and mental did a lot for the dissipation of my depression. This exercise was one of my three umbilical cords that led to my sanity. Faith and spirituality resulted in the publication of eight books of my creative writing: collections of poems as prayers. Exercise both mental and physical freed my mind from that which depressed me.

Another umbilical cord that was most significant was my prayer life. It is my faith that is my lifeline. Joan and I used to pray together before her cognitive impairment made her unable to do so. Now, I just recite the prayers to her that she once knew so well. She is comfortable and at peace because of that, even though she doesn't remember a few minutes later. I am okay with this because I know that God will listen to her prayers if she was able to pray herself, and her comfort in listening is prayer enough for God.

When I take her to church she will say the prayers like the *Lord's Prayer* quietly. Evidently being in church, hearing others praying the same prayer involves Joan's long-term memories that were rooted in her mind so many years ago. Numerous aspects of religious tradition and practice invoke in Joan memories of familiar prayers, rituals, and hymns. I feel that these religious practices are deeply rooted in the memory portion of Joan's brain. The depression seems to lift from her when she is in the pew praying and singing with others. Her singing is flat and monotone for she doesn't remember the melody.

But to me it doesn't matter because it is a manifestation of a quality of life that has remained. The organized structure of the church service has a familiarity for the person with AD.

These sorts of small victories—no matter how short lived—will help me as a caregiver with my depression. The Catholic Mass is especially good for the AD patient because its predictable structure is the same the world over even though the language spoken is not the same. The music that is played in the church can evoke long-term memories. Spiritual singing in a traditional church setting can be therapeutic to the AD patient and it surely was in Joan's case.

I knew that Joan liked big band music. She liked the big bands of Glenn Miller, Tommy Dorsey, Jimmy Dorsey, Harry James, Benny Goodman, Harry James, and Cab Calloway. I had big band music in our collection of CDs, especially of the WWII years. Big band music of the 1940s and 1950s she loved. I played this kind of music to Joan with headphones over her head. She would move her hands, her legs and her entire body, jiving with the music. I became a firm believer in music therapy. There was no indication of depression when she listened to music. Consequently, my own depression dissipated, and this enabled me to do creative writing and especially spiritual poetry. This made me feel good and the sense of accomplishment brought a feeling of exhilaration and peaceful joy to my own mind.

Anger in Alzheimer's and Depression

Every so often Joan would get angry and direct her anger toward me, because I was usually the only one present and the fact that I had corrected her on something and gave a directive for own safety. I had to be forceful in my instruction, in order to keep her from involvement in a high-risk situation. For example, she has a bad habit of pulling at her hair. She has done this for three years. She gets angry at anyone who asks her to stop doing that, whether it is me or someone else. In her anger, she will use swear words that she has never used before her AD. Joan has thrown things at me. She picks up anything within reach and throws it. This action is always directed at me.

One time she threw a portable CD player and it is a delicate instrument. Fortunately, it survived that harsh treatment. At times, in her anger at her AD condition, she tells me that she wants to die and she wishes she could do it. I have seen Joan angry at anyone who tells her not do something like the hair pulling. If I try to get her to eat some of her food she gets angry. It doesn't take much to tick Joan off.

I learned that feelings of anger and depression with the Alzheimer's patient will give way to denial of the reality of memory loss. This condition occurs in the second stage of AD where cognitive impairment is not acute. What I learned from my experience with Joan, and from the residents of *Autumn Hills Alzheimer's Care Facility*, is to my keep voice gentle and to use diversion tactics when I encounter anger in someone with AD. I use few words, but with lots of inflection. Fortunately for the AD patient, the angry incident is quickly forgotten, but the caregiver remembers it with pain, though also with forgiveness.

When I first observed anger in Joan, I was hurt because she was taking it out on her caregiver who gives her everything so that there is some quality to her life. I learned that anger is a symptom of AD, and that it can be both passive or very aggressive. I thought she was very self-centered and that everything revolved around her needs. I learned that this is a common occurrence with people with AD. Joan's anger appeared in the second and third stage of AD. As of the writing of this book, Joan has not exhibited violent aggression. Joan prior to her AD was a gentle and altruistic person.

Alzheimer's and Illness

One Friday afternoon I found my wife Joan in the lobby of the *Autumn Hills Alzheimer's Care Facility* shaking uncontrollably. She was cold and had no use of her legs. I was afraid she was having a stroke. The nurse on duty didn't see signs of a stroke, but nevertheless advised me to take Joan to the emergency room of the hospital. I chose the emergency room over a prompt care facility, because I was familiar with it and the competency of the medical staff there. With the help of the nurse and an aide we placed Joan into my vehicle. We managed to put her in the front seat because her immobility required the space it afforded. I drove quickly to the hospital emergency room (ER) and derived assistance there in getting Joan out of the car and into a wheelchair. Once inside we registered and were taken to a room with a clinical setup. Joan was undressed and put into the infamous hospital dressing gown. She was placed on a table and immediately an IV was inserted as well as a heart monitor. The insertion of the IV needle caused Joan to recoil and scream out in pain. She never has acted this way before. It took the nurse several tries before the needle was in place. Blood tests were also taken and again she recoiled with screams of pain. Her sensitivity to pain was increased manifold. A heart monitor was attached to one of her fingers. Joan immediately tried to shake it off.

Joan did something that she never did before the onset of Alzheimer's disease. She tried to remove the IV from her arm and at the same time attempted to shake off the finger sleeve. She was angry and confused. I talked to her in a calm tone, stroked her face and told her it was going to be fine. The diagnosis was that Joan had a severe urinary tract infection. For four hours I stood alongside her examination table and kept vigil on her attempts to remove the lifesaving umbilical cords. Her anger rose to a high level as a nurse constantly controlled her hands and arms so the contact points would not be dislodged. Her anger was directed to me because I was the one she thought was responsible for what she considered restraints. At least this was what it appeared to be to me. Her being an AD patient compounded the difficulties encountered in the ER examination room. It was a nightmare for me as a caregiver. She was not following any directions at all. This I understood was to be expected of AD patients. I used soothing words, I maintained a calm tone, and I tried distraction. None of these worked with Joan because I felt the noise outside of the examination room was distracting. I turned to prayer said aloud and I held both Joan's hands in mine to restrain her movements. I prayed over her the familiar prayers Joan and I would pray together. They were the prayers we would recite during our vespers reading and also during the church services. I prayed the Rosary (for we are Catholic). I used a variation of the Rosary where we pray for individual family members and friends on each of the beads. Joan closed her eyes and her lips moved in synchronization with my words. Eventually she went to sleep.

After five hours in the ER we were taken to the 3rd floor of the hospital and placed in an assigned room. The IV and the heart monitor were exchanged for the ones already in the room.

Joan slept the entire night and dinner was not eaten nor available. Joan was not ready to eat in her present condition. She was receiving electrolytes and antibiotics as well as other medications through the IV. Joan also slept through the entire next day and was only awakened to eat meals, use the portable toilet, and to take medications. Her legs were shaking and she could not stand unassisted. She needed to be manipulated in changing position and getting in and out of bed. It took two aides to help her with the basic daily needs. It was the next day where Joan repeated the behavior she exhibited in the ER. It was a daylong vigilance on my part to keep Joan from setting off all the alarms associated with the monitoring devices. At one point, she became extremely angry and attempted once again to remove her IV and heart monitor. She sat in a chair for the entire day. Boredom and immobility played havoc with Joan. Every time she tried to arise from the chair an alarm would go off and Joan would get angry. She told me that I didn't love her anymore and why was I keeping her restrained. There was an excellent physical therapist who worked with Joan in using her legs to get out of the chair and walking short distances. The occupational therapist was also excellent. Much of the occupational therapy was also physical therapy. Joan did remarkably well after the therapy sessions. On the morning of the fifth day of the hospital stay we were discharged from the hospital.

I would like to recoup what I have learned from illness with someone who was in the hospital and has AD. Especially from hospitalization for one experiencing Alzheimer's disease.

1. Always be ready to make the AD patient safe and comfortable. Have something warm to put on them if they are cold. This also holds true when the AD patient is being transported.
2. Establish good means of communication. This is especially true in communication with hospital staff.
3. Never have more than one person giving directions. This adds to the confusion for the AD patient, because it is difficult for them to assimilate directions.
4. Get the AD patient's attention before giving commands or directions.
5. Always assume that the present behavior can be altered by the illness.
6. Sensitivity to pain may be enhanced.
7. Always use the patient's first name when addressing the AD patient.
8. Place your hand on the shoulder, back, or arm when establishing confidence, especially in terms of body support.
9. It is good to use nonverbal clues. The AD patient will respond to hand gestures or smiles, or clapping of hands, or thumbs up when something is done relatively well.
10. Communication difficulties may be the greatest challenge for the caregiver and this is intensified by the illness.
11. Be gentle in moving the hospitalized AD patient. They will experience discomfort and may resist or yell loudly with the pain of movement.
12. Keep reminding the AD patient where they are and where the bathroom is located.
13. Accentuate your approval when a task is accomplished.
14. Never do a task yourself, but seek the help of a hospital staff member such as a nurse or aide.
15. The hospitalized person with AD needs to be happy with a feeling of intimacy with the caregivers from the hospital.
16. Establish a line of communication between you as the major caregiver and the hospital personnel.
17. Remember that the patient's inability to think logically and understand practical problems does not improve with a change of environment, but is in fact intensified by it.
18. Spatial relationships will inevitably change with location change.
19. Remember that the AD patient is still the same person who left the health care unit to go to the hospital to get well again.
20. Illness may increase the level of depression, because of the added burden of the illness.
21. Maintain your own level of happiness and optimism and convey it to the AD patient and the hospital staff.

Visits to hospitals need not be traumatic for the AD patient. Keeping a person happy and active should be a priority, whether at home, in a healthcare facility or in a hospital. The illness needs to be cured and the AD patient needs to feel well, for the burden is heavy even without adding to the burden by hospitalization. I hunger for the life I used to have. I will never experience that life completely ever again. Whether the burden is lifted from my shoulders or whether it remains for an indefinite length of time, I am forever changed. Caring for someone with AD is still a responsibility that I accept.

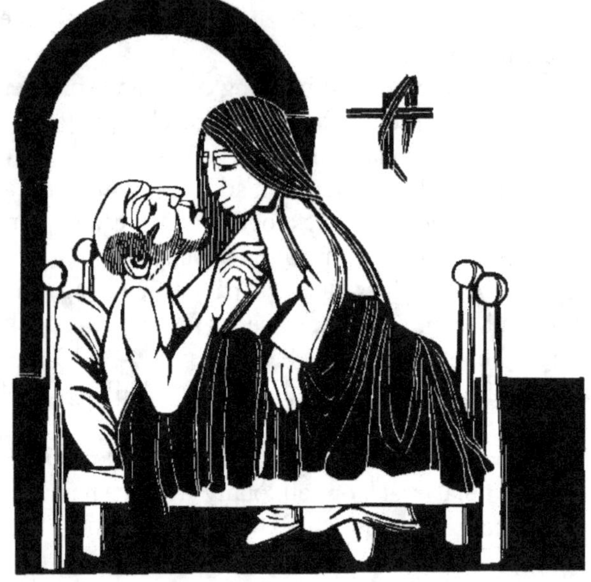

Care for the Caregiver

Taking care of myself as a caregiver is probably one of the most important things that I could do for my wife. If something happens to me—and it eventually will happen—who is there to take care of Joan? My family members all have jobs and lives of their own to lead. They do what they can when they can. My daughter-in-law who has been of exemplary help should not be saddled with the care of her mother-in-law. She has other sets of aging parents who may require her support. The ultimatum for me is to take the best care of myself that I possibly can for as long as I can. I am the one who is primarily responsible for a loved one with AD, and it is essential that I take care of myself while caring for Joan for her sake and mine.

What I do to cope with stress and depression is to use three things:

First, I exercise doing both aerobic activity and weight resistance activity. This is easy for me to do because I love to exercise. I enjoy the high I get when the endorphins kick in. Because of my military accident I have exercised since I was twenty years old almost every single day, no matter where I am. My injury was spinal related and the Air Force doctor assigned to me recommended exercise over invasive surgery. I have blessed the accident for it was the catalyst for my good health over the years.

Second, I am a creative writer. I have written books of poetry, books about the environment, books on spirituality, and articles both in the environmental education field and in the field of the enhancement of spirituality. I can reach out with my creative writing umbilical cord to the world outside of my caregiving world. It relieves any stress or depression that I might have because of my caregiving responsibilities. As of the writing of his book, I am learning to speak the Italian Florentine dialect instead of the southern dialect that I already speak.

Third, are the hobbies and interests that I have. I enjoy outdoor photography and often go afield to capture wildlife with my camera. I enjoy fishing, and particularly fly fishing. It is when I am standing in a mountain stream, fishing for trout, that I am completely happy and at peace. These types of outdoor recreational activities are always accessible to the caregiver who may be locked into a home environment unable to travel.

Some of the things that I have learned as a caregiver for over four years are listed below as tips for the caregiver. By definition, a caregiver is a person who helps the person with AD without being paid to do so. Most often it is a spouse or an adult family member. The caregiver is the key individual involved in the care of an Alzheimer's patient.

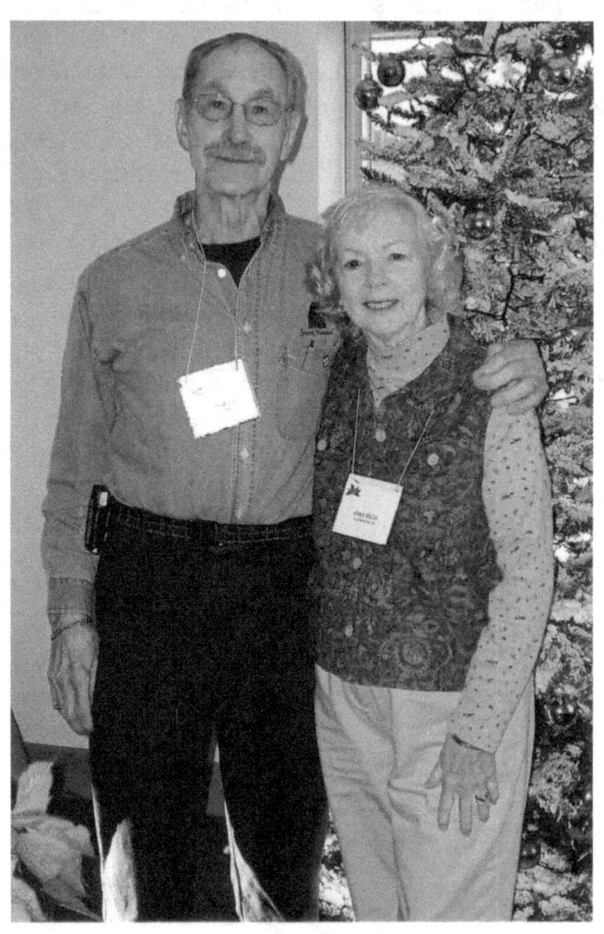

Tips for the Caregiver

1. Recognize early the behavioral changes in the person you care for
2. Learn to recognize the difference between dementia and AD
3. Learn the seven stages of AD and recognize the symptoms in each stage
4. Continue to learn more about AD
5. Overcome denial of AD by the caregiver and family members
6. Develop coping strategies with health professionals
7. Consider joining a support group
8. Learn what strategies are available to caregivers
9. Involve others when insisting on activities for a person with AD
10. Allow others to help you, the caregiver, with your responsibilities
11. Provide firsthand experiences for those who volunteer help
12. Do not always expect family members or friends to help with caregiving
13. Look for help in those who are compassionate, altruistic, and loving
14. Realize that AD is progressive, and plan for institutional care
15. Do not wait until there is dire need for outside help
16. Realize that the challenges inherent in care of AD patient will intensify
17. Remember that AD will change a person's outward behavior
18. You, as a caregiver, need to recognize the need of taking care of yourself
19. Recognize the incidence of burnout and seek help
20. The caregiver's life and that of the person with AD are greatly intertwined
21. Engage in socialization activities. This is vitally important
22. Recognize that, as AD progresses, so do the challenges to the caregiver
23. Caregiver should engage in physical exercise as well as mental exercise
24. Do some aerobic and weight resistance exercises as time permits
25. Maintain a healthy diet for both caregiver and person with AD
26. Address anger and/or depression which may manifest itself in the caregiver
27. Work on increasing the level of patience when dealing with a person with AD
28. Never shout at a person with AD. The patient often perceives it as threatening
29. A caregiver's voice commands should be calm, soft, gentle and well modulated
30. Always keep your AD patient in safe environments
31. Remove all dangerous items from the AD patient: things such as knives, poisons, etc.
32. Always present a jovial mood and good humor to the AD patient
33. As a caregiver always have joy in your heart and hugs in your arms
34. Building a support system is an important step in seeking help

Note: There are so many other things that a caregiver can do. The above tips are gleaned from my experience both in caring for Joan and the time I spent in *Autumn Hills Alzheimer's Care Facility*. Living with AD patients gave me insights into the progression of AD. Progression is a word that best describes what I witnessed when spending seven hours a day at the care facility.

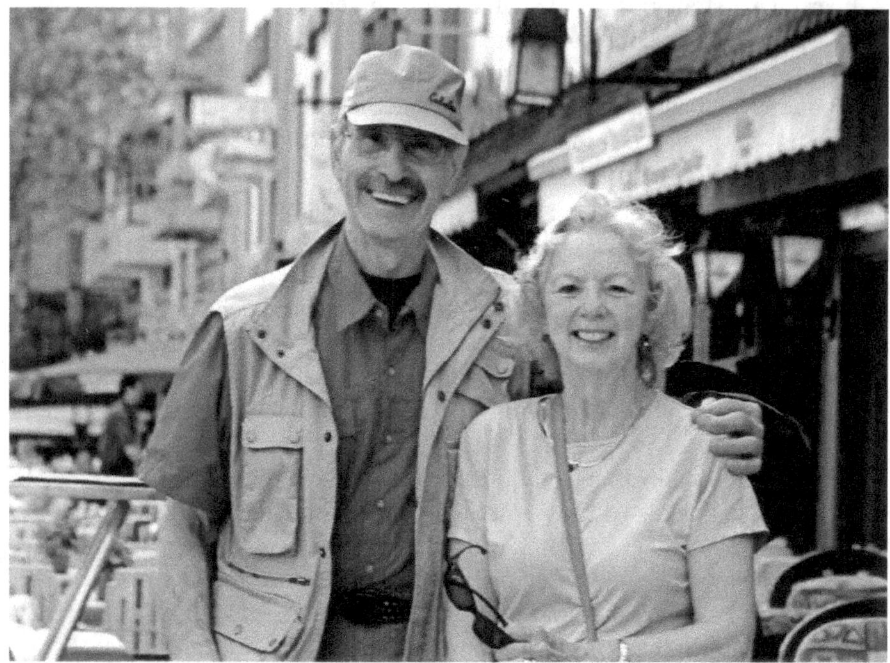

Part 2:
Insights into Alzheimer's and Caregiving

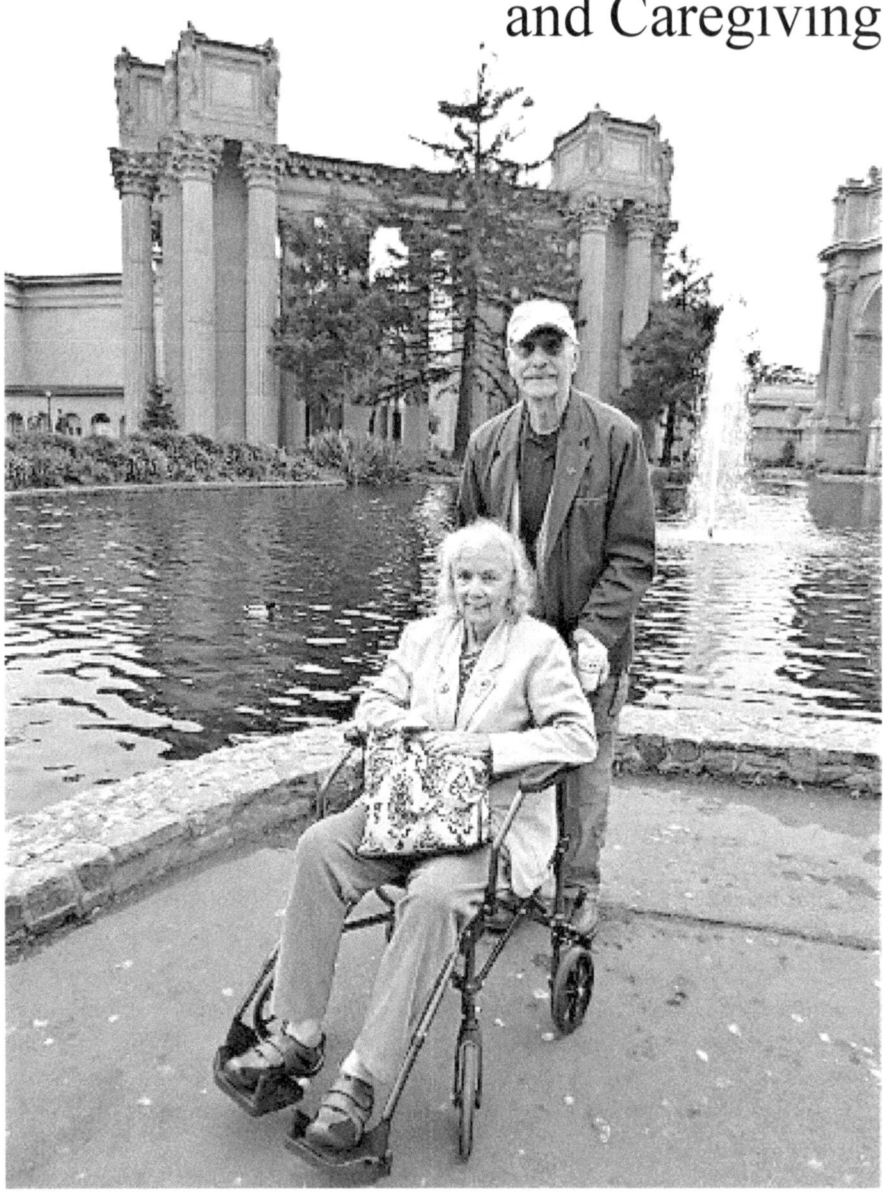

Reflective Thoughts on Caregiving

Note: I wrote this article when I first cared for my Joan during her early stages of Alzheimer's disease. It refers to my emotional thoughts about something I thought I would never have to do. My Italian mother said to me when I was a young adult: "Tommy, marry someone younger than yourself and she will take care of you in your old age." Well, it didn't work out that way. I married someone seven and a half years younger than I, and here I am caring for her because of AD.

I never could have conceived that my golden years would be my tarnished years. My wife Joan fell victim to the horrible disease known as Alzheimer's. I am seven and a half years older than Joan. The first stage of this disease begins as dementia and lasts for approximately three years. My life began to change as the demands of caregiving began to increase. I am approaching my ninetieth birthday and my body meets the daily challenges of total caregiving with less strength and endurance each passing day. What I miss the most is the socialization that I used to have. I feel that I am a prisoner in my own home. I am anchored in place by my caring responsibilities. We used to be a team with each of us sharing the responsibilities of maintaining a household. We are no longer a team and I do everything including the daily maintenance of Joan. It has been said that you do not really know someone until you walk a mile in their footsteps. The same thing can be said about caregiving. You never know what it is like until you experience it 24/7.

Each day is the same and so very repetitive. It is this repetitiveness that gets me into a depressed state myself. My wife's needs come first, and my own secondary. I pray each and every night and day for my patience to not lessen. After all, this is still my wife even though she acts differently, and I must remember her love and unselfishness over the many years of our marriage. I sincerely feel that marriage is a holy covenant and the vows that I said at the marriage ceremony are to be taken seriously. This commitment and prayer sustain me most of the time. But there are times when I simply want to run away from it all.

Experts on Alzheimer's say that the first three years is where recognition of loved ones disappears. It is at this stage where I feel Joan will accept outside help in the form of someone who is not immediately known to her. It may even mean institutional residency.

Family members and friends tell me that I should take care of my own needs to stay healthy both physically and mentally. Sometimes caregivers die before the individual they are caring for. In my case the differential in age may be the case. In this case, the love of my family members will prevail, and they will exercise good judgement. Some have given me resources to explore and alternatives to pursue as the disease progresses. This I accept and I will continue to read and listen.

I fully realize that I cannot continue to do it all by myself. I have had some help from my family members. However, they do have active lives to lead, and should not be encumbered by additional time and energy, absorbing responsibilities for aging parents. It is so hard to let go of someone you have loved and still do. We have shared so much over sixty years. It is so difficult to relinquish caregiving to others who do not have the same love, no matter how professional they are as caregivers. Until the threshold between dementia and Alzheimer's is fully crossed, and recognition is gone, then outside help will have to be initially of at-home variety.

I fully realize that Joan is still that wonderful person inside the same body. Only her memory has changed her outward personality. A terrible aspect of the disease is the memory loss. All the memory of our experiences both as family and in the experiences of raising our children is gone. I attempt to relive these experiences for her, but I know that she will not remember what we shared together over the years. My heart breaks when I see the loss of a sharp mind in a woman of so much talent and cognitive skills.

I ask God: "Why have you treated one of your most loyal servants with such a debilitating disease in her old age?" I am not angry with God, but I am disappointed. I know that in His infinite wisdom He has a reason for our situation. But I have yet to discern what that reason fully is. Can it be that He is testing me or punishing me for my past sins? I do not think God would do that. If anything He would punish me, and not Joan. I know one thing for sure. It is that I have grown stronger with regard to humility and patience. Even though at times I just want to throw up my hands in defeat, I swiftly realize how wrong that would be. I know that my prayer life has grown in intensity and scope.

I must overcome my loneliness and lack of socialization. It is difficult and very challenging for me to do so. But do it I must. Each day I die a little bit more. The death is manifested more in a mental state than a physical one. I know that I am baring my inner soul and heart when I write about reflecting on total caregiving for a loved one. I am not writing this for sympathy, but rather as an umbilical cord to a world that I loved. My love for Joan has to be stronger than that external love.

I know God has blessed me with many gifts among which is my creative writing which serves as my conduit to the outside world. I have written spiritual poems and published them. Eight volumes of collective poems representing over 800 poems. I have also written books and articles on Benedictine spirituality. I hesitate to think the loss of Joan's brilliant mind is a high price to pay for this conduit to the outside world. She sleeps to midday and gives me time to do all sorts of required tasks. I think the most difficult thing to fully accept is the loss of a very cognitive mind. So I pray often during the course of the day and night. My insomnia allows ample time for prayer. I will do all that I can to ensure that everything is done to make Joan comfortable and to monitor all medications including alternatives.

These reflections are not meant to be lamentations. Perhaps other caregivers can profit from my experiences. This is the price humanity has to pay as lifespans extend.

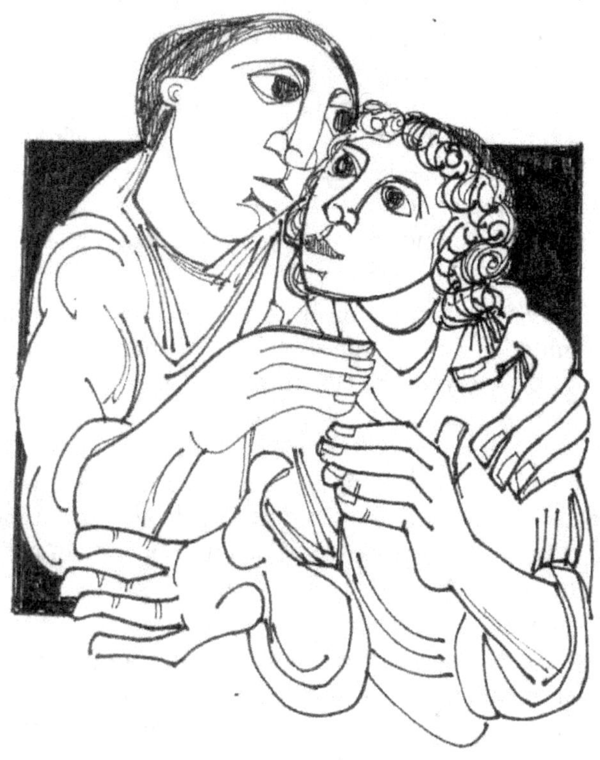

Resources Helpful for Understanding Alzheimer's

In the last five years, resources for caregivers of AD patients have dramatically increased. Most helpful to me were the TED talks on Alzheimer's. These talks are short, but most informative. One of the talks that was a catalyst for me in defining AD was the talk by Lisa Genova. She is a neuroscientist with a doctorate degree from Harvard University. I used the TED app both on my iPhone, iPad and my home computer. Dr. Genova states that Alzheimer's doesn't have to be the destiny of the brain. In her talk she shared the latest science investigating the disease.

She shared with the listener some promising research on what one can do to build a brain resistant to AD. For me her talk defined what AD is and what we can do to slow it down. She concentrated on the synapses in the brain. There are trillions of synapses in the brain. When we learn something new we add a synapse. Learning Italian, meeting new friends, reading a book, are some of many activities that will add to cognitive reserve. One study involving 100 nuns all over the age of eighty-five showed no signs of cognitive impairment. They were all well-educated and were constantly learning. All the nuns donated their brains for research. Although they had amyloid plaque clogging the synapses, they showed no visible symptoms of AD.

This helped me understand why my wife Joan had no sensation of a bowel movement, or sense of taste, or no sense of smell. From this talk I learned that sometimes the synapse begins to break down from within, especially when choked with amyloid plaque that begins to bind, creating what is called tangles. Dr. Genova talked about the importance of deep sleep where synapses are repaired or new ones added. She said in her talk to think of a seesaw and when early symptoms of AD begin to tip the scale. Something like cardiovascular disease, genetic inheritance, obesity, diabetes, can all tip the scale.

Although Joan is well past the early stages of AD, the information I gleaned from Dr. Genova's talk was helpful to me as a caregiver. It gave insights into the nature of the disease. Dr. Genova said that the slowing down of Alzheimer's will lie in the development of preventive medicine and keeping the transmitters from being blocked by the clogging of the synapse by attacking the amyloid plaque. She also alluded to the fact that an early diagnosis fifteen to twenty years before the early symptoms of AD will prolong the advent of early symptoms of AD. She advised the early use of the PET scan. The diagnosis doesn't not mean death before it is time. I also found her book: *Still Alice* to be a valuable resource. It recounts the experience that a professor had when diagnosed with Alzheimer's when she was in her mid-fifties. The book has been made into a movie using the same name. It can be viewed on *Netflix* or *YouTube*.

Another interesting TED talk was the one given by Samuel Cohen. He titled the talk: *Alzheimer's Is Not Normal Aging and We Can Cure It.* He begins by stating that more than 40 million people worldwide suffer from Alzheimer's disease, and that number is expected to increase drastically in the coming years. But no real progress has been made in the fight against the disease since its classification more than 100 years ago.

Samuel Cohen, a scientist shares with the viewer a recent breakthrough in Alzheimer's research. The research is ongoing in his lab. Cohen states that AD is a disease and we should treat it as such. He also says that we can cure it. Cohen referred to Dr. Alois Alzheimer who was treating a patient who was taken from an asylum and placed under Alzheimer's care. This was in Germany in 1901. Her name was Auguste Deter and she was very symptomatic of this brain disease. She died in 1906. Dr. Alzheimer was given permission to do an autopsy on Auguste Deter's brain. What Dr. Alzheimer found was a brain the likes of which he had never seen before. That was 114 years ago. In all that time, very little research was even attempted to find a cure for Alzheimer's disease. Cohen stated that this was due to a lack of awareness. There is much more funding for research in cancer, cardiovascular disease, and HIV. In the age group 85 or older one in two individuals will have AD.

As I researched AD, I found many organizations helpful in providing more information. I found their websites, and contacted them via the internet asking for information about AD. One very good resource was *The Alzheimer's Association*. This voluntary organization, based in Chicago, coordinates the efforts of over 100 chapters in the United States, promotes changes in public policy and funds research. The website provides helpful information and can link one to chapter websites. Especially helpful to me were their numerous publications and reading lists.

The *National Institute on Aging* was another organization that was very helpful to me as I coped with my caregiving responsibilities. The Institute provided me with many free publications that helped in understanding AD and how to cope with caregiving challenges.

Alzheimer Web (WWW.alz.org) was a very useful resource for me as I sought to understand Joan's AD. This was one of the first websites devoted entirely to AD. It provided me with up-to-date information about medical advances about caring for someone with AD.

Another source of AD information was the magazine publication *WebMD*. It frequently had articles pertaining to dementia, memory loss and AD. This magazine, which appears in any doctor's waiting room, is free.

In it, I found an interesting reference to new research on AD. It was entitled: "The Tao of Tau". A major focus of Alzheimer's research is to find a way to detect the disease before irreversible brain damage occurs. Tau protein builds up in the brains of people with Alzheimer's but is difficult to test. Chilean researchers have now devised a test that can detect plaque in blood platelets. A study of 53 people with Alzheimer's and 37 healthy people confirmed that those with Alzheimer's have higher levels of tau in their blood.

The researchers hope this could lead to a simple inexpensive blood test for earlier diagnosis. This article first appeared in *The Journal of Alzheimer's Disease*. This journal is another resource for understanding AD.

Much too late for Joan, but of interest to caregivers of AD patients, are the very first symptoms of AD. The May 2017 issue of *WebMD* had an interesting short clip on music therapy for AD patients. It was entitled: "Sound Mind". It opened by saying, whether you prefer country, rock, classical, or hip-hop, music is good for the brain. Many of us know the feeling we get when we hear a favorite song or medley. We have a undeniable urge to move our feet, tap out the rhythm, or even burst out in song. According to Stephanie Watson, "music has a powerful ability to improve mood, especially when we engage in it."

A film resource presents music as therapy for the mind. The film *Alive Inside* is an excellent resource for learning how music therapy can improve memory if only for a little while. The film opens with an African American elderly man sitting in the dozing, head-slump posture. Headphones are placed over his ears and immediately his eyes open wide and he sits up straight in his wheelchair and says out loud: "Cab Calloway, I know the man." He starts moving his feet, tapping on the wheelchair arm rests and starts what is called in the vernacular "jiving".

I have used music as therapy for Joan to some degree of success. She jives with the big band sounds of the forties, fifties, and sixties. It seems to make her more relaxed and in a happier mood. She has less stress hormones when she listens to music from her past. She seems to be aware of who and where she is.

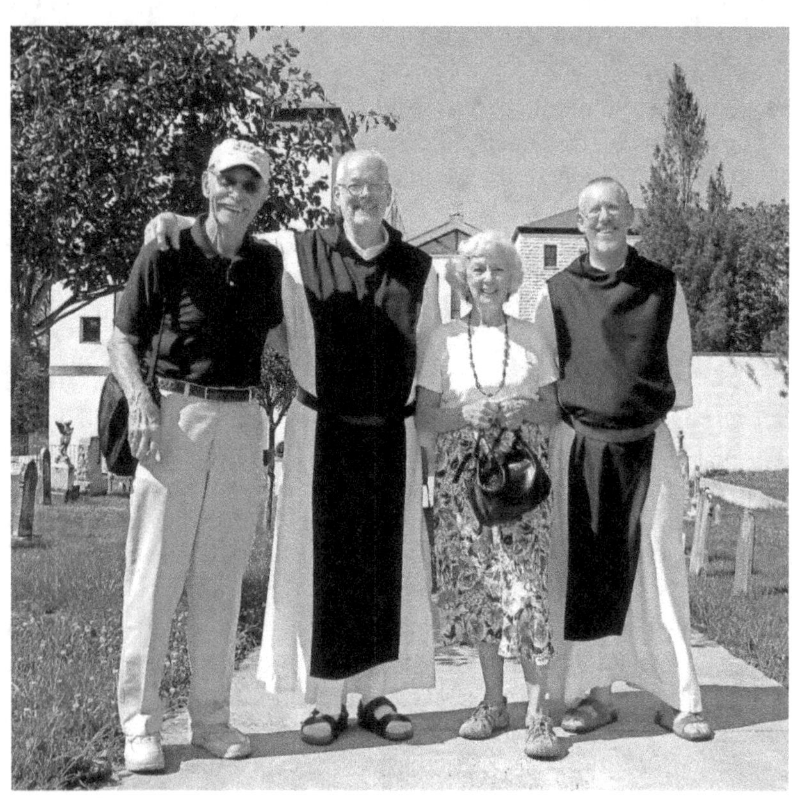

My Spirituality Is My Lifeline

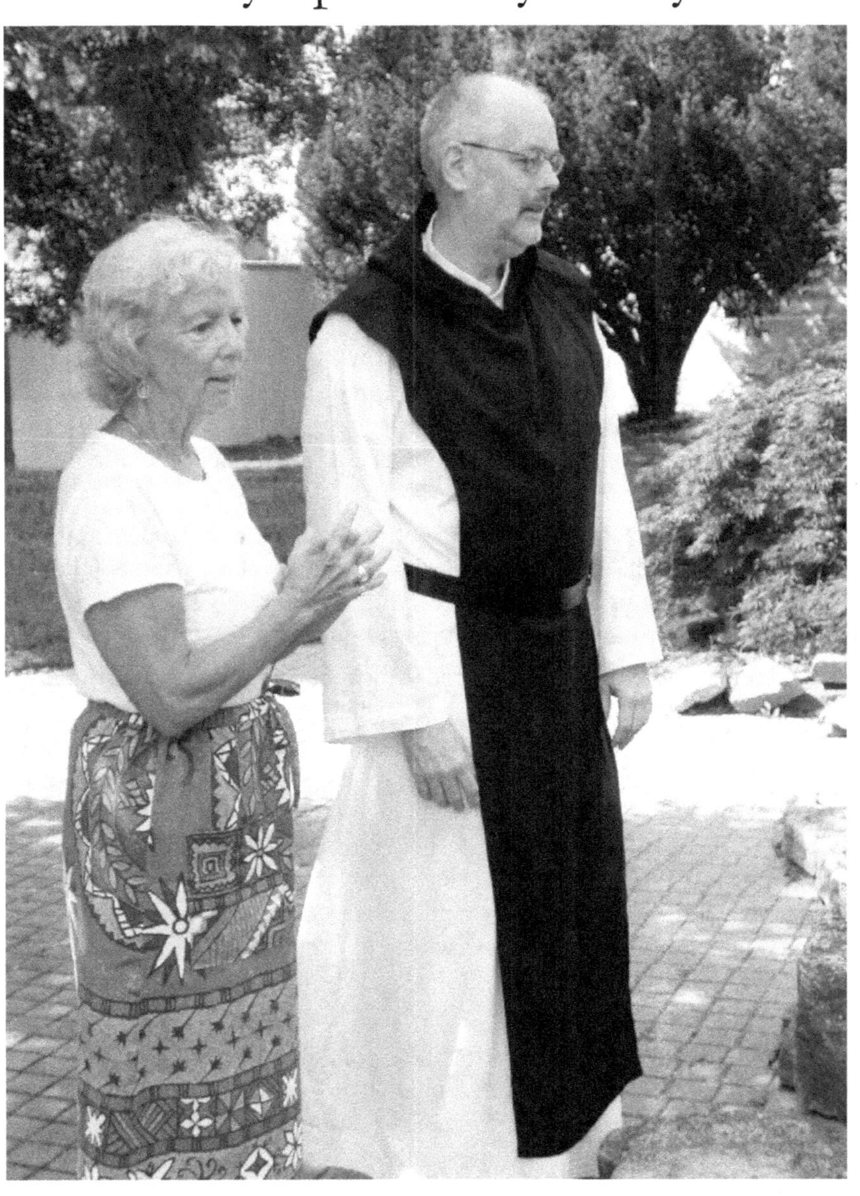

My Spirituality Is My Lifeline

I am compelled to include how spirituality has been my lifeline in coping with Joan's Alzheimer's disease. A lifeline is defined by me as being a supporting rope, keeping me alive and bringing me to safe shores. This is what caregiving feels like. The responsibilities and challenges are overwhelming. I felt like I was drowning in a body of water and a rope was thrown to me. That rope drew me onto terra firma or firm soil. My feet are solidly planted on a supportive surface. Physically and emotionally I was severely challenged.

The analogy here is akin to stepping into a body of water and not knowing how to swim. You do not know at the outset how deep the water is or how turbulent the water is. This is the same situation as when a caregiver first assumes care for another individual. It is true especially when the person cared for has AD.

Prayer has been a life-enriching experience for both Joan and me. Unfortunately, Joan cannot remember how we would pray together. Spirituality is a broad term and not always understood. I was not always a very spiritual person. However, life experiences such as several near-death events have awakened in me that someone greater than I was looking out for me.

Getting married to Joan provided more reasons to become a spiritual person and to establish a relationship with God. Now I had someone other than myself to pray for and with. We both were of the same faith. This helped a lot when our family began to grow in numbers.

I am an oblate of Saint Meinrad Archabbey in St. Meinrad, Indiana. The word oblate refers to the middle ages when nobles and the rich wanted their sons to be educated beyond just a rudimentary education. The most learned individuals were found among the ranks of monks living in monasteries. The nobles or rich fathers would pledge their sons to the monks to be educated. A gift of money was most always promised by the parent of the boy to be given over to the monks. The monks accepted the child in hopes that, upon reaching adulthood, it would elect to remain in the monastic community and be a monk. Today we pledge ourselves to pray like the monks and abide by the Rule of St. Benedict. My wife Joan is also an oblate of Saint Meinrad Archabbey.

Nothing ever prepared me for the rigors and trials of caregiving. In my golden years, I have been given a challenge by God to express my love and care for someone who is undergoing memory loss. It is called Alzheimer's disease. It was both physically and mentally stressful. I had to adjust to living a life that has completely changed from what it once was. I had to give up many activities that I dearly loved. Proclaiming the readings for Mass as a lector was a hard one to give up. My volunteer work at the YMCA, where I was a physical rehabilitative trainer for seniors was another.

My traveling on pilgrimages with Joan, my wife, was especially difficult to curtail. Giving up my writing for the Benedictine Oblate newsletter was also hard to accept, although I continue doing so from afar via the computer. Most of my social life became nonexistent.

The question that I had at the outset of Joan's AD was: "How do I retain my sanity through the repetitive caregiving tasks that I do every day?" I did these caregiving tasks 24/7. First is my love of my spouse, and equally my love of God and His son Jesus. My faith journey had to be strengthened. I had to decrease so that I could increase.

My marriage is a contract or a spiritual covenant. "For better or worse, till death do you part" were powerful words that implied an unwavering commitment. I hold the vows that I spoke as sacred vows never to be broken. This did not change in its implicit application toward the challenges of total caregiving. It is one of the most challenging commitments I have ever had to make. My faith in God and my subsequent prayer life, augmented by my Benedictine oblation, have been a saving grace.

My prayers ask God to give me the patience that I need in my caregiving responsibilities. This is where the vow of humility has helped me to achieve a level of patience that I was previously not endowed with. The vow of silence has helped me to sustain gentleness involved in listening. That my spouse was saying "I cannot remember" had to be heard with understanding. Obedience to the basic rules of caring for someone with memory loss emanated from my Benedictine oblation and the acceptance of the vow of obedience.

The *Liturgy of the Hours* or *Divine Office* has been a healing grace. My wife Joan and I once read the inherent prayers together. Now I pray the *Liturgy of the Hours* by praying it aloud to her or just by myself when she is sleeping. Excessive sleeping is a characteristic symptom of AD.

My Benedictine oblation and my writing for the Saint Meinrad Archabbey community have augmented newfound time to be creative. The loss of a beautiful mind has been heartbreaking. This has been difficult to accept. Stepping up my prayer life and faith journey has helped a great deal.

The change in my lifestyle has been difficult to accept. The only constant has been my prayer life, where the routine rituals dovetail nicely with my caregiving routine. This is where my Benedictine oblation has been so valuable in keeping me on course in caregiving.

God has shown me that love for another person and the care of that person are gifts from Him. It has been said often that to give up one's life for that of another person is the highest expression of love. As a Benedictine oblate, I find that it is very natural to apply humility to my caregiving situation. The promises of silence and obedience have been equally of value. I open each day with saying: "O Lord, open my lips and my mouth shall proclaim your praise." He is testing my marriage covenant every day. He is also testing my covenant to Benedictine oblation and its inherent spirituality.

Note: Parts of the above treatise appeared in *Benedictine Oblate*, Winter 2016, Volume 22:1.

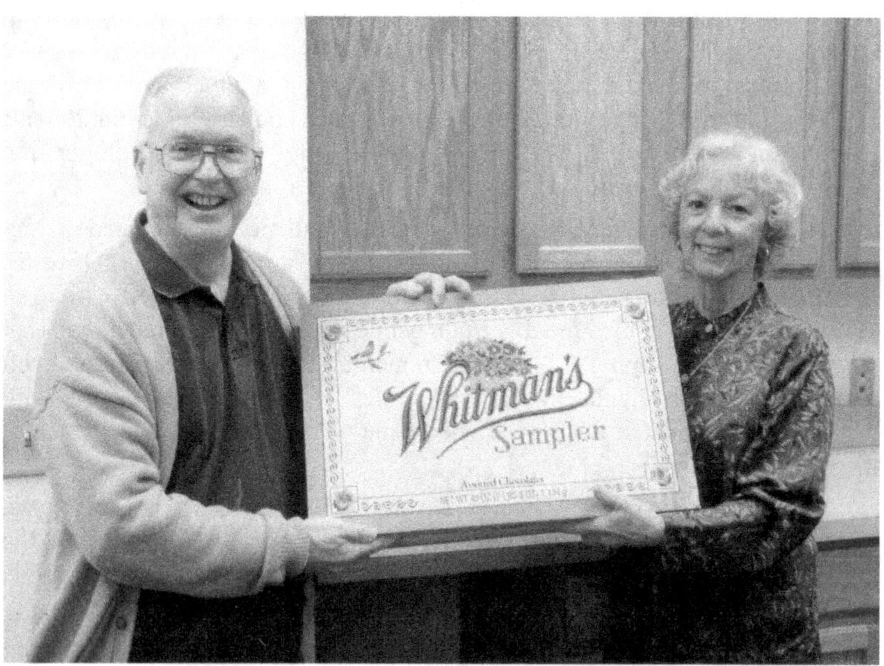

Part 4:
Quotes that Foster an Understanding of Alzheimer's

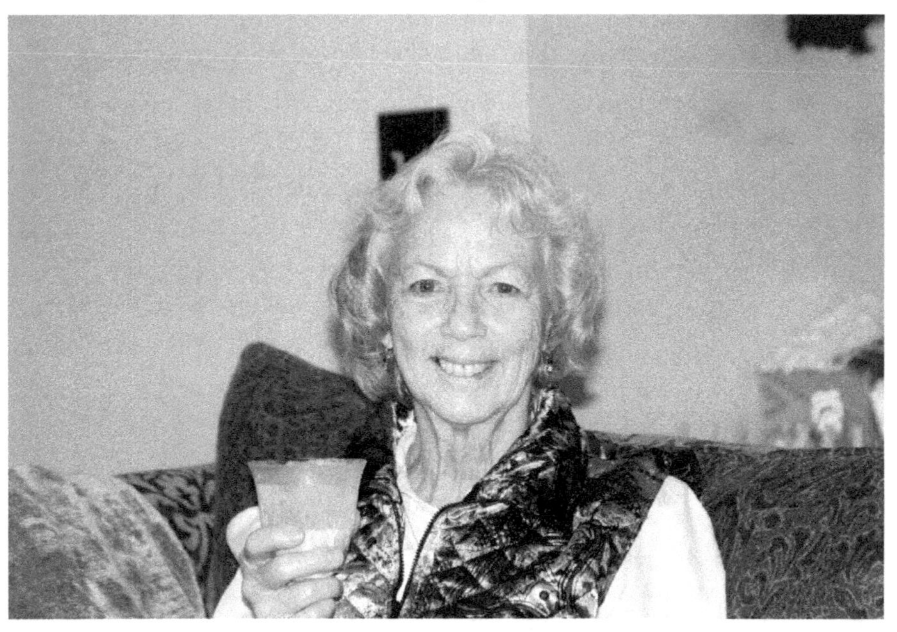

Quotes That Foster an Understanding of Alzheimer's

The following quotations are the ones that gave me hope, optimism, joy, and courage amid my challenges as a caregiver for someone with AD. It is hoped that perhaps these quotes will help the reader who also may be a caregiver.

Even though the flame is no longer visible there is still life in the embers.
— Thomas J. Rillo

Common sense and a sense of humor are the same thing, moving at different speeds. A sense of humor is just common sense dancing. — William James

Mirth is God's medicine. Everybody should bathe in it.
— Henry Ward Beecher

You have to leave the city of your comfort and go into the wilderness of your intuition. What you will discover is yourself. — Alan Alda

It is evident that we are dealing with a peculiar, little known disease process.
— Alois Alzheimer

I have recently been told that I am one of the millions of Americans afflicted with Alzheimer's disease. — Ronald Reagan, President of the United States

Your life is a gift from God. What you do with that life in the service of others is your gift that you give back to God. — Thomas J. Rillo

What you leave behind is not etched in stone monuments, but rather it lives on in the minds of those you have loved. — Pericles

Marriage is a covenant or a sacred contract. The vows pledged in the marriage ceremony are sacred and serious and they should never be broken.
— Thomas J. Rillo

As we cultivate peace and happiness, we also nourish peace and happiness in those we love. — Thich Nhat Hanh

When you look at your life, the greatest happinesses are family happinesses.
— Dr. Joyce Brothers

We cannot live only for ourselves. A thousand fibers connect us with our fellow-men. — Herman Melville

Music washes away from the soul the dust of everyday life.
— Berthold Auerbach

Talk about things from the past. Recent memories will fade more quickly.
— Kristen Cusato

Every day is a new day. A bad day yesterday does not mean a bad day today. Take it one day at a time. — Kristen Cusato

I have found the paradox that I love until it hurts, then there is no hurt, but only more love. — Mother Teresa.

You can't live a perfect day without doing something for someone who will never be able to repay you. — John Wooden

All movement is life. If the brain can tell the legs to move, you will slow down the infirmities that accompany the aging process. — Thomas J. Rillo

Physical exercise and mental exercise can slow down the progression of Alzheimer's. — Thomas J. Rillo

We can do no great things, only small things with great love.
— Mother Teresa.

Never judge a book by its cover. So, don't judge a person by their outward countenance. You first open the book and read the pages and so it is with the AD patient. — Thomas J. Rillo

Wife is a verb not a noun. It implies movement dedicated to the care of family, friends and those in need. Now is the time for a caregiver to be the movement. — Thomas J. Rillo

Alzheimer's is a disease, not an infirmity. Recognize that it is and proceed accordingly. — Thomas J. Rillo

Humor is just another defense against the universe. — Mel Brooks

It ain't over until it's over. — Yogi Berra

The highest reward for a person's toil is not what they get for it, but what they become by it. — John Ruskin

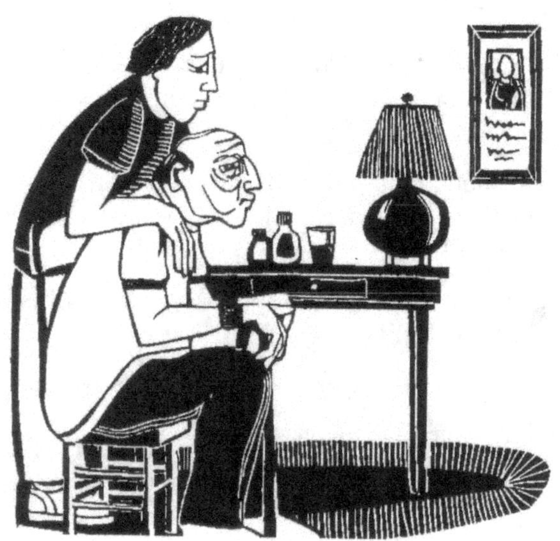

Part 5:
Poems Influenced by Joan's Alzheimer's

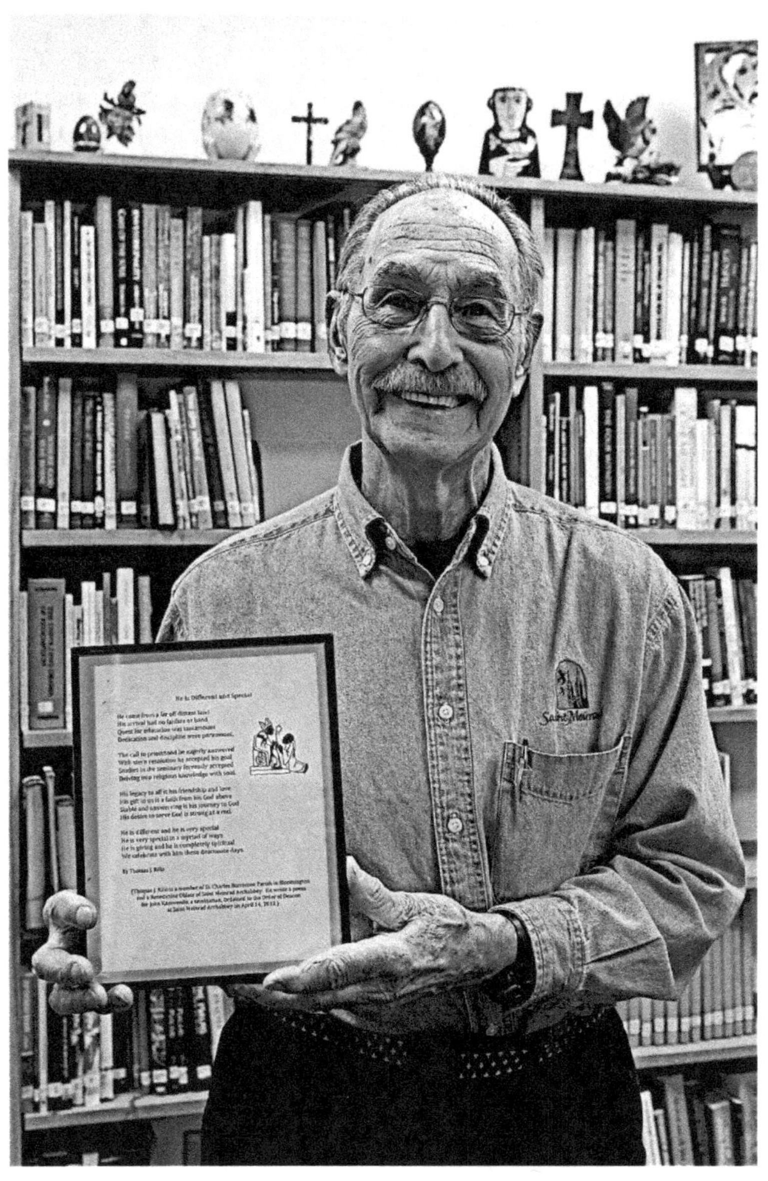

It took an unbelievable number of years for a river to carve out the huge chasm known as the Grand Canyon. Our lifespan is so very short in comparison. We have our memories of our visits to this grand natural feature. Unfortunately, even these memories are short lived for some as disease steals the memory. However short the memory, the essence of it remains somewhere in the recesses of the mind. — Thomas J. Rillo

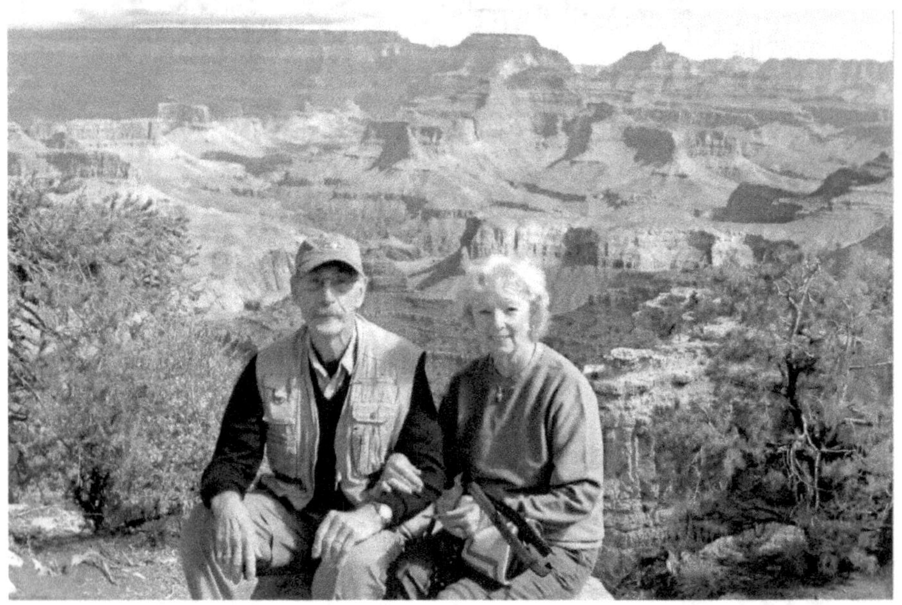

Poems influenced by Joan's Alzheimer's

I am a poet and have published eight books of spiritual poems. This book on caregiving for Joan represents what I have experienced and learned from association with AD. I could not resist inserting some poems about my living with a person who has AD

During my caregiving time, I had the opportunity to create poems about AD. Joan's progression with this horrible disease inspired me to write poems about how AD changed our lives. This I chronicled via poetic format. I do not intend to castigate either Joan or other persons with AD. They are the victims of this insidious disease and they did not choose memory loss. I admire their courage and their tenuous hold on what remains of their former lives. AD patients or people with Alzheimer's are my heroes. My association with them during my hours spent at *Autumn Hills* made me love every one of them and taught me, however inadvertently, a pragmatic definition of AD. This has made me a better person. Caregiving for Joan also made me a better person. In times of war there is no greater sacrifice than to give up your life for another. This is the way it is for the caregiver. We volunteer with love in our hearts to do gentle caregiving and sacrifice our lives for our loved ones. Enjoy the poems and see if you, as a caregiver, can find yourself in the poems.

Note: All the illustrations are by Br. Martin Erspamer, OSB. Br. Martin is a monk of Saint Meinrad Archabbey in St. Meinrad, Indiana. Br. Martin is an acclaimed artist of liturgical art. His speciality is the creation of stained glass windows although he is also creatively active in a wide range of art including ceramics, pottery, painting, sketches, drawing, water color, oil painting, etc. Br. Martin has a legendary reputation throughout the art world. The author is indebted to him for the generous contribution of his art work in many of the author's previous books.

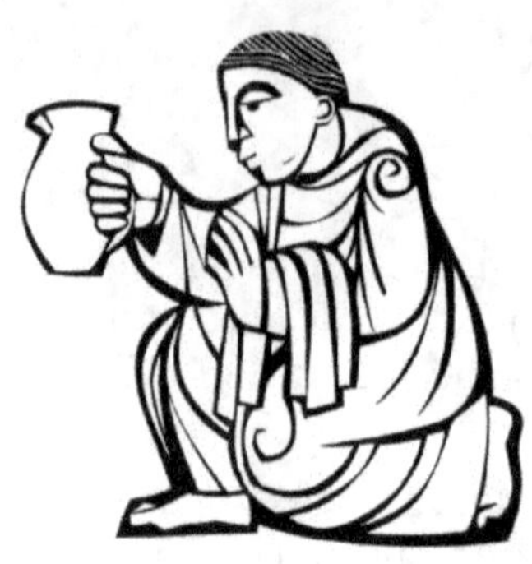

A Caregiver's Journey

Unless you walk completely in a caregiver's footsteps
You will never fully know the full scope of challenges
The day by day routine of caregiving is overwhelming
The stress and strain of doing everything for an AD patient
     A caregiver's journey

It can be so unbelievably stressful when coupled with other tasks
The stress of watching a loved one's memory slowly slip away
The heartache keeps pace with the progression of memory loss
You look up at heaven and ask the proverbial question "Why, God?"
     A caregiver's journey

You watch attentively the progressive stages of AD disease
You grieve for the beautiful person within who is also beautiful externally
Yearning to share memories of the good times experienced together
Memory of the experiences shared together cannot be remembered
     A caregiver's journey

Day by day you live with your loved one with a horrendous monster
You feel powerless to stop the progression of this consuming disease
You do what you can to make the loved one safe and comfortable
Examination of the quality of life will be an indication of letting go
     A caregiver's journey

Guilt will raise its ugly head and totally consume the caregiver
Support groups are fine and work to some degree but the guilt remains
Guilt becomes a part of the caregiver's persona from the onset of the disease
The saving grace is that it is not a question about you, but about the AD patient.
     A caregiver's journey

A Caregiver's Prayer

I pray that my faith in God will always sustain me
      Sustain me in my new role as a total caregiver
That God will give me the gift of loving patience
      That previously I was not overly endowed with
I pray fervently that our love for one another.
      Will endure all the hardships as it once did
When we were first married, it was enough
Then disease manifested itself
Any plans for living were drastically altered
      I was frightened that I could not measure up
To the myriad tasks that we once both shared
      I ask God to help me with the heavy burden of care
To give me the strength to withstand the challenge of rituals
      The bombardment of repetitive situations
The disease doesn't lessen the reality of her existence
      I pray God continues to extend my gifts of care
That He speaks to me, for I feel often that I am alone
      Especially the gift of His sustained love for me
That God grants me stamina, patience and understanding
      To always have faith that the Holy Trinity will be with me
Understand my life changes having faith in God's plan
      For a marriage is a covenant with many promises to keep.

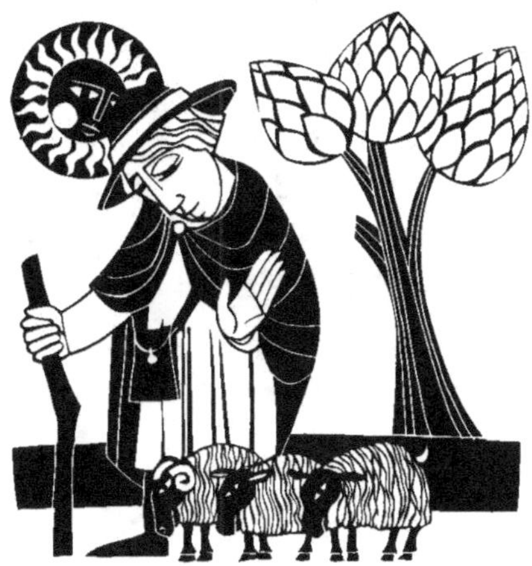

Asleep on the Outside, Awake Inside

Memory loss is an abyss of aging
It manifests itself inside the brain
Cognition is often very depressing
It progresses slowly like a freight train

Progression of the disease moves slowly
Balance becomes unbalanced with time
Depression is frequent when one is lonely
Appetite lessens and no desire to dine

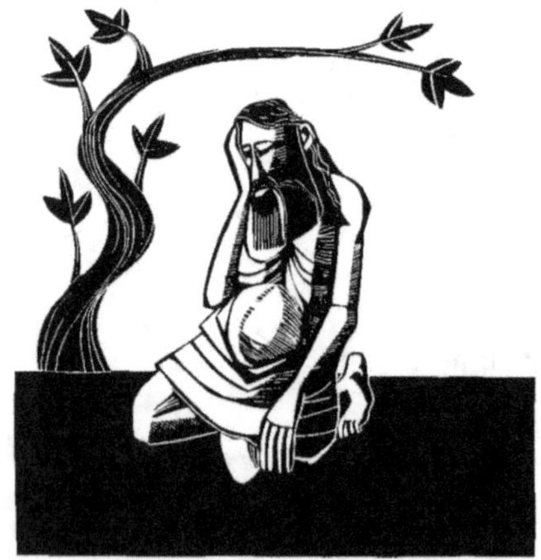

Sleeping at odd times is common
No interest in activities that require cognition
Common grooming requires a care person
Mobility necessitating assisted action

There is the same entity within the body
Communication is difficult and words fail
But it is the same person that is embodied
It is analogous to that person being in jail

With severe loss comes sleep on the outside
Very much alive is the same person within
This doesn't imply that personality has died
Instead it means to use techniques and begin

The axiom to remember is easily applied
That the person is alive on the inside
The same person is asleep on the outside
Reach the inner person with restraints untied.

Caregiving Is a Challenge

Nothing has prepared me for this challenge
Caregiving is indeed a serious challenge for me
I am sustained by my love for my spouse
Sustained also by my faith in God the Father

My life has changed radically in a myriad of ways
Socialization has been reduced to a bare minimum
It is as if I am a prisoner in my own home
My sanity is maintained by the love for my faith

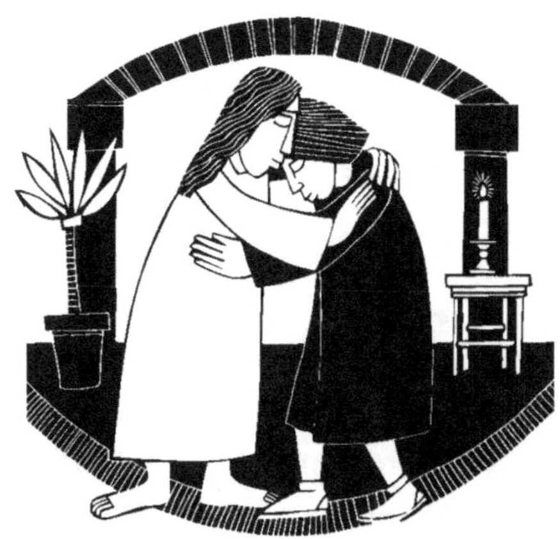

Marriage is a contract or a loving covenant
The vows spoken in the marriage are sacred
They are to be heard with ear of the heart
Not to be broken under any circumstances

It is not easy to be a caregiver, but it is rewarding
It gives a sense of meaning of what it is to be human
The greatest gift that one can make is to sacrifice your life
Caregiving is akin to laying down your life for another life

Without faith through prayer I could not survive
I need to decrease my own desires and increase
Increasing in honing the caregiving gifts God has given me
I cannot do it alone without God's unconditional love.

Caregiving Is Not a Sprint

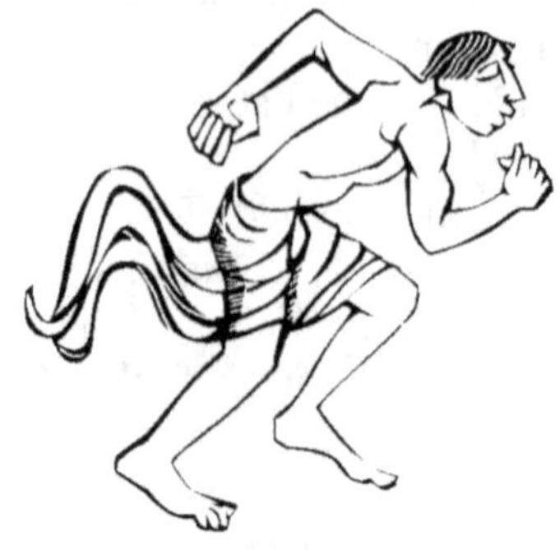

Caregiving is not a sprint but a marathon
The multitude of tasks involved are repetitious
There has to be something that stabilizes sanity
Confinement and loss of socialization is manifested
          Caregiving is not a sprint

What sustains a caregiver in staying with that task
Of giving what had been a life to care for another
Love for the one being cared for can be one variable
Faith in God that bestowed the responsibility is another
          Caregiving is not a sprint

The disease of memory loss proceeds ever so slowly
It extends over a long period of time in marathon length
Prayer and spiritual application can be the soothing ointment
Faith in God that will make the obstacles lessen in severity
          Caregiving is not a sprint

Frustration can be a debilitating factor for depression
Why did God place on me such an awesome burden?
His message that I decrease in order to increase I hear
That I would be a better person because of my caring load
          Caregiving is not a sprint

Coping, Always Coping

Adversity that never lessens
Challenges that always confront me
Caregiving continually tests me
When can I lay my head down

Is God punishing me for my sins?
Sins forgotten but not by Him
What will support me in my trials?
Love and faith in you my God

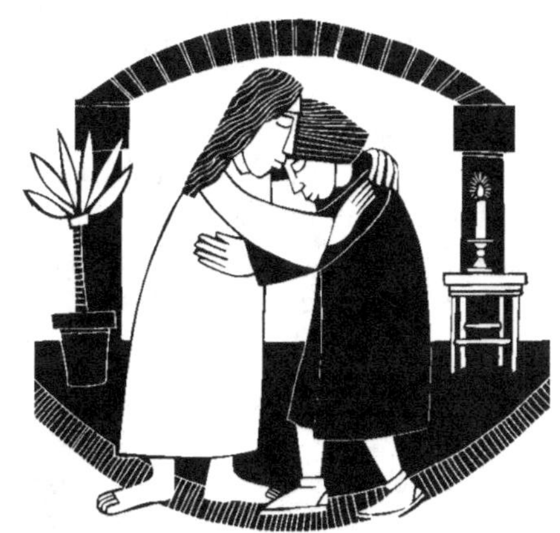

Will sustain me and support me
The monotony and routine depress
My umbilical cord to you is prayer
Prayer the soothing balm for stress

Hear me as I reach for your embrace
Coping, alway coping with spousal needs
The horrible monster Alzheimer's raises
Its ugly head to manifest in the brain

It descends heavily upon my spouse
Every day she slips further away from me
Shared memories begin to fade away
They are accessed only in my mind

The joy of shared memories vanishes
The recalling is only with my framework
Does God want me to be stronger?
Stronger in caring, giving, and loving

In altruism is found my true strength
To know the time for letting go
To let go and to let God.

Faith Helps with Caregiving

There is no greater challenge than that of caregiving
It is a profound life-changing experience for the caregiver
You give of yourself and how God helps you to grow
Grow stronger in love, patience, gentleness and humility
      Faith helps with caregiving

We think of our memory as that what defines us
It gives us continuity, a history instead of a collection
A collection of disparate impressions that are useless
Unless you have dementia or Alzheimer's disease
      Faith helps with caregiving

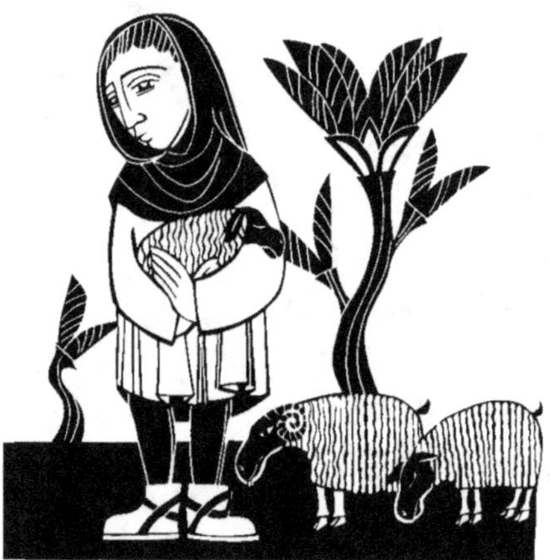

You care for a person because of love and compassion
You lay down your life and socially die for them in care
It is a twenty-four seven-day commitment you accept
Knowing that the person you care for is the same person within
      Faith helps with caregiving

What is it that sustains us and nourishes with hopeful energy?
It is through our God-given faith in prayer that we keep our sanity
We pray with our loved ones even though retention is not there
We persevere because God and Jesus are there to hold us up.
      Faith helps with caregiving

Letting Go

The hardest decision I have ever made in my entire life
Was when because of Alzheimer's disease
We, as a family admitted Joan their mother and my wife
Into an Alzheimer's Care Facility although she was displeased
      Letting go

Sixty years of marriage that included four years of care
Made it extremely difficult for me to let her go
Gone was the intimacy and closeness we always share
It was for the best we were told by those in the know
      Letting go

The nights are very lonely times for me
I reach across our bed and she is not there
As I wander through the house many signs of her I see
Without her I am so lonely an emotion I cannot bear
      Letting go

Oh God, why do you let this happen, this insidious disease?
Allowing it to run amok among the elderly stealing their identity?
Is Alzheimer's a penance or a challenge for me to seize?
I struggle with the wisdom of my decision and feel guilty
      Letting go

I let go of my beautiful wife to the care of professionals
Knowing that it is for the best is not the expected solace
I acclimatize to the situation and keep up my morale
I ask God for strength with my caregiving and to bless us with grace.
      Letting go

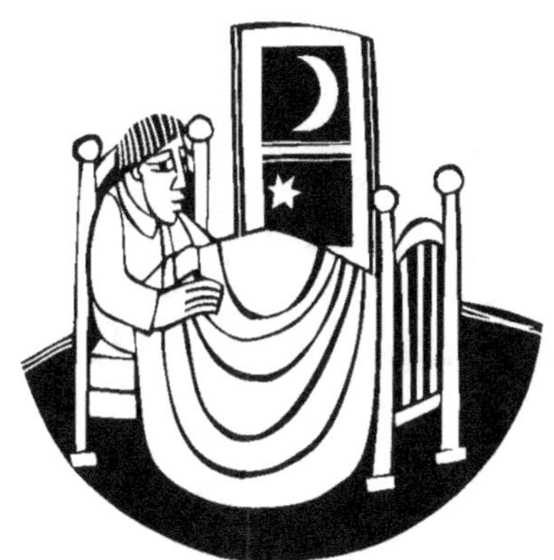

Life Is Like a Glowing Ember

Life burns until it is an ember
With flames flickering with life
With more flames, it constitutes one life

Now the flame flickers
Much like a life when memory fails
Loss of movement a flame flickers
It is akin to a human life

That burns until it is an ember
Once a vibrant life
Similar as losing familiar words.
Searching for words

To complete thoughts
Recalling recent experiences
The ember still glows but slowly fades
It is the progression to a coal

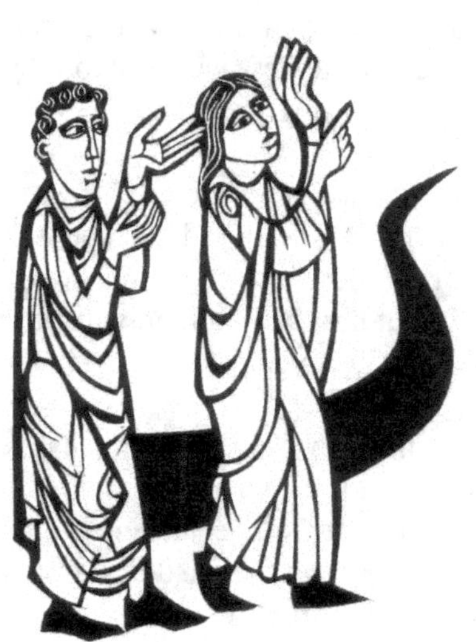

Culminating in death
Nothing can breathe life into it
A person with Alzheimer's disease
Mirrors the progression of a dying fire

Memory loss and dementia
Like the flames that burn up the fuel
It becomes coals, embers and ash
Once the match is lit the flames consume

Once AD is diagnosed the progression begins
No cure as the hands hold back the clock
No optimism or hope
The warmth of the fire fades

The warmth of the persona fades
For as long as an ember glows
There is hope for rekindling the flames
If only for a short while

Only God can blow out the fire
We let go and let God.

Music, a Therapeutic Gift from God

For the cognitive disabled individual music has therapeutic value
    The music bypasses the mind and enters the soul
Their hands move and their feet tap rhythmically
    Their hands move in cadence with the melody
Music, a therapeutic gift from God

Mouths lipped the words remembered from long ago
    If the music represents songs from their cognitive years
Then remembering is added by familiar songs of their youth
    Memory games such as remembering the band or singer
Music, a therapeutic gift from God

Finish the title when just a few words are the clues
    Agitates unused memory cells in recognition of the lyrics
Reminiscing bypasses the brain and moves into the soul itself
    The need for music as a therapeutic tool with memory loss
Music, a therapeutic gift from God

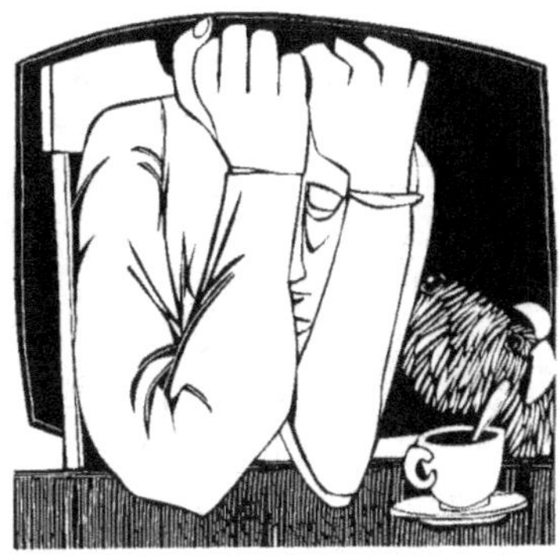

Invaluable in slowing the horrible disease called Alzheimer's
    Recognition that there is a life still within the body
Is a critical first step in caring for the individual with severe memory loss
    The reaction of the afflicted is evidence enough for music therapy
Music, a therapeutic gift from God

Let us bring those minds back to their enjoyable younger past
    Wheelchair-bound individuals with memory loss can dance
Square dance a natural for the application of music to movement
    There is still an ember within the sleeping mind
Music, a therapeutic gift from God

The ember needs to be kindled for a spark of life quality.

Oh Lord, Why Am I Alone?

After sixty years of marriage you took my spouse away
       Not physically but mentally she left my side
Proclaiming that I was an awesome caregiver they say
       How could I be anything else, for I love my bride
Oh Lord, why am I alone?

I watched the horrible disease lay claim to a brilliant mind
       Slowly year by year my spouse began to slip away
Marriage is a Holy covenant and vows said tightly bind
       I take them seriously and I remain faithful to this day
Oh Lord, why am I alone?

Now my spouse is admitted to an Alzheimer's care facility
       We are separated for the first time after sixty years together
It was the hardest decision I have ever made in the face of disability
       I return to our home every evening to be alone and it is not better
Oh Lord, why am I alone?

Loneliness is a two-edged sword cutting relentlessly every night
       I look up to the heavens and I ask: "Oh Lord, why am I alone?"
I examine my situation and ask why has God punished me with all His might
       Is it a punishment for my past sins that He wants me to atone?
Oh Lord, why am I alone?

No, it is God's will for me to grow strong in the face of adversity
       To exercise my faith and to believe in Him and in His wisdom
He answers my prayers with something better for my spirituality
       I am alone because God wants me to be ready to enter His kingdom
Oh Lord, why am I alone?

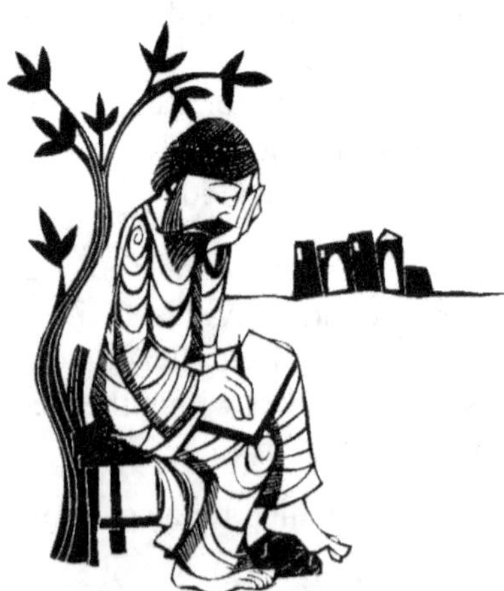

Still Joan Inside

My spouse's name is Joan
Named for Joan of Arc
A strong-willed woman
Who lived in France
Champion of inalienable rights
Both for women and for men
This was Joan on the outside
And also vocal for human rights
Kindness and selfishness
Both external and internal
A robber baron descends
A robber baron called Alzheimer's
It begins to steal away memories
Synapses begin to clog
Joan gropes for words
Words to fit thoughts
Fear descends shrouding the brain
The fog of depression tries to rise
Joan tries ever so hard
To vocalize her thoughts
Her brain cannot breach
The impediment to her speech
The original Joan resides inside
Residing inside she is alive
She has lost the rational path
Her sense of wonder fades
The cloud of sadness is perennial
I am her caregiver and spiritual guide
I am her umbilical cord to God
I am her prayer leader
Until such time I let go
I let go and let God.

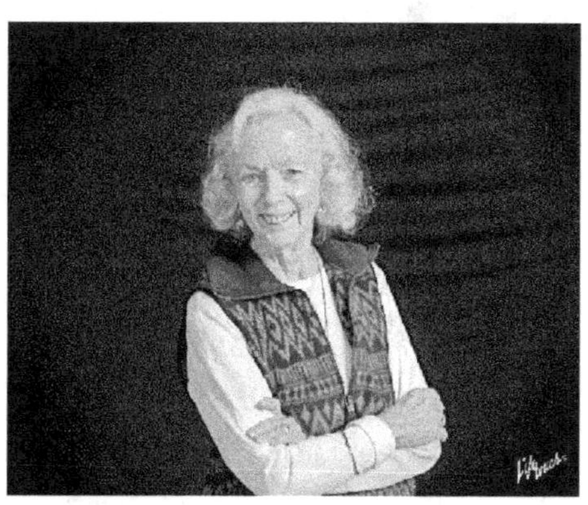

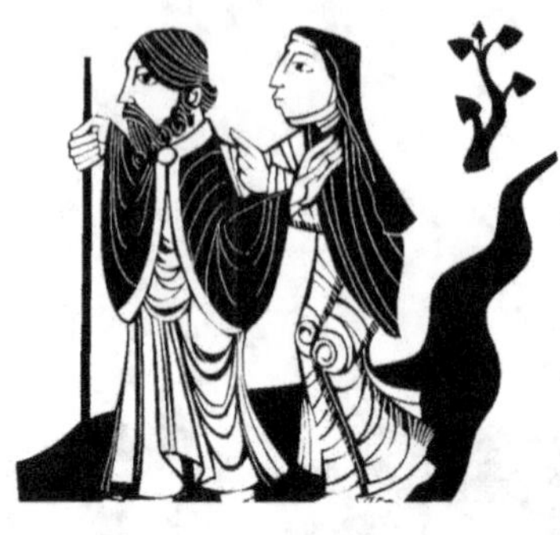

Two Lives Diverged

Two lives bonded and welded by Holy matrimony
    Sixty years of familial union with one partner
Accepting marriage as a sacramental covenant
    Vows taken years past still valid and adhered to
Two Lives Diverged

The marriage journey was not always a smooth course
    Talking and communicating leveled the bumps
Similar faith an asset to problem solving in harmonious union
    Placing family members before self accepted by both
Two Lives Diverged

Travel memories began to accrue and wonderful to recall
    The sharing of exciting times traveling the world
Reminiscence as a life-enhancing activity in senior years
    A monster of a disease raised its ugly head and lives changed
Two Lives Diverged

We both did not choose our senior years harnessed by this disease
    I, in the knowledge of what is happening, endure the pain
The mantle of memory loss is like a protective blanket
    It erases all knowledge and even awareness of what is happening
Two Lives Diverged

One life is totally absorbed in caregiving responsibilities and challenges
    The second life is internally withdrawn into an impregnable shell
Protected by a shield of memory loss that wards off stress and anxiety
    Two lives diverge and continue their journey to God on separate paths.
Two Lives Diverged

The Tragic Loss of Memory

The tragic loss of memory
>Memories should remind us of good times

Of all that has joyously gone on before
>Memories of loved ones and of special friends

Some of whom have passed and we see them no more

The tragic loss of memory
>Memory loss is an obstacle to recollection for two

Memories are to be shared with loved ones
>A horrible disease of the mind erases all

It is sad to witness it and makes loved ones so blue

The tragic loss of memory
>Memories remind us of places we will never see again

Wonderful new travel experiences cannot be recalled or shared
>In old age memories are all that one can enjoy in reflection

The condition of a loved one causes the caregiver much pain

The tragic loss of memory
>'Why does God let this happen?' one might fervently ask

Is it because He wishes for memory loss to soothe all pain?
>It is a penance extended to loved ones and caregivers

Lifespan is much longer and some with memory loss live only in the past.

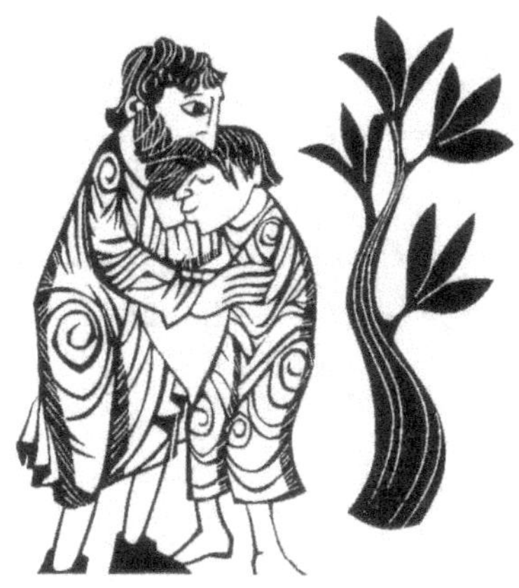

Why Does God Allow This?

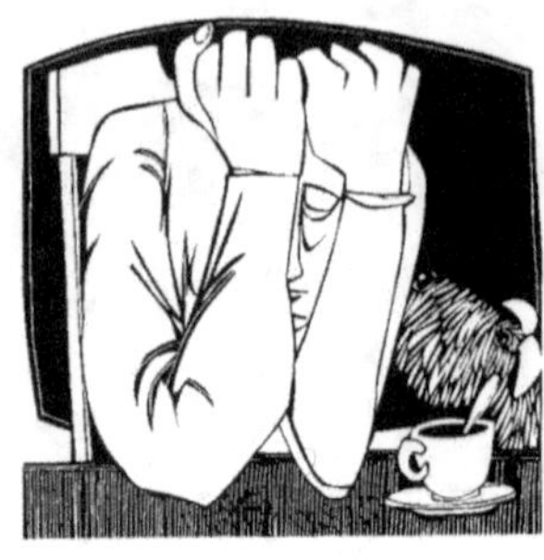

Why does God allow this?
For the aged there is a horrible disease that can happen
Modern medical advancements have increased longevity
With advanced age comes a severe memory loss condition
It is called Alzheimer's and more women than men have it

Why does God allow this?
Research has not found a remedy for this progressive condition
Individuals who formerly led productive lives are drastically changed
They are the same person in the same body but with decreasing cognition
Caregivers are taxed to the limits of their physical and mental support

Why Does God allow this?
One asks why does God let this happen to individuals who are good?
What is God's rationale for allowing this undignified journey to happen?
We know that we cannot fathom the mind of God and we can only guess
There has to be a reason for pain and suffering that happen to good people

Why does God allow this?
We can only speculate and assume that family members grow stronger
In caring and loving those with severe memory loss, they grow in strength
They become more altruistic and with unselfishness serve loved ones
We see changes in individuals who care for victims of Alzheimer's

Why does God allow this?
In the caregiving support lifestyles are changed and sacrifices made
God lets pain and suffering happen to the caregiver in their responsibilities
We can never know the mind of God nor can we fathom His decisions
The strength comes to the support individuals who care for those afflicted.

Why Does God Let This Happen to Me?

Why do you let this hardship of mine be such a burden?
I know that I need to bear its weight with acceptance
Acceptance that is fueled by my love and faith in you
The total caregiving that I administer is diminishing me
I want to scream and run away from it all
My penance I feel is far too long in duration
The years pass by and my responsibilities increase
The former strength of my body weakens with age
What keeps me from giving up and running away?
Spousal love is the catalyst for my continual commitment
Marriage as a covenant binds me to my marriage vows
The routine of total care emotionally drains me
But the umbilical cord to my sanity is my faith
Prayers are the emotional balm that eases mental pain
Even though the subject of my caregiving cannot absorb
I remember our marital commitment to each other
I must diminish myself and accept why God has allowed this
I need to relinquish my guilt and seek the help of others
Others who care about me and see the pitfalls of total caregiving
God has let this happen to me for a reason He deemed best
It has made me stronger as a husband, and in my faith
I keep to the routine of daily prayer even though I pray alone
My affiliation with my church and monastic community is my rock
Without their prayers and support I would sink into an abyss
I put my trust in my God and know that His judgement is fair
Only He knows what His design of my continued life will be
His voice is clear and strong as I listen to the wisdom of His words
Just knowing that He loves me and is with me always
It is enough to give me the strength I need to persevere.

The strongest and most enduring survival unit on earth is the family.

The family united in love and support can endure almost any disaster, cataclysmic event, discriminatory and prejudicial action, and economic chaos.
— Thomas J. Rillo

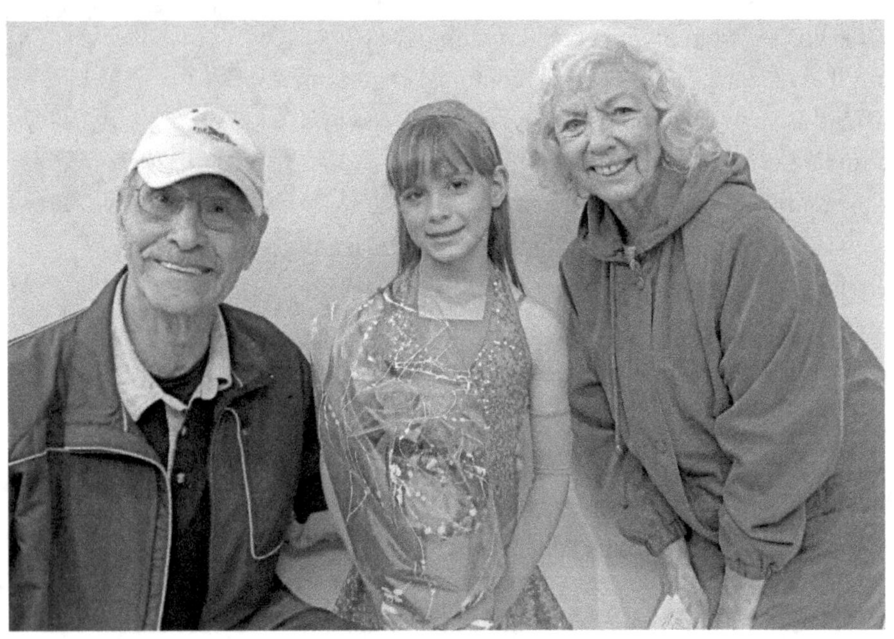

References

Genova, Lisa. *Still Alice.* New York: Pocket Books: Division of Simon & Schuster, 2009

Mehlinger, Howard D. *Caring for Carolee: What It's Like to Care for a Spouse with Alzheimer's at Home.* Bloomington, Indiana: Author House, 2014

Newmark, Amy & Angela Timashenka Geiger. *Chicken Soup for the Soul: Living with Alzheimer's & Other Dementias.* Chicken Soup for the Soul Publishing, LlC, A Joint Project with the Alzheimer's Association, 2014

Kuhn, Daniel. *Alzheimer's Early Stages: First Steps for Family, Friends and Caregivers.* Alameda, CA: Hunter House Inc. Publishers, 2003

National Institute on Aging. *Understanding Alzheimer's Disease.* Publication No. 15-5411, October, 2015

National Institute on Aging. *Understanding Memory Loss.* Publication No. 15-5442, October, 2015

National Institute on Aging. *Caring for* a *Person with Alzheimer's Disease.* Publication No. 17-AG-6173, January 2017

Smith, B. & Gasby, Dan. *Before I Forget.* New York: Harmony Books, 2016

Family

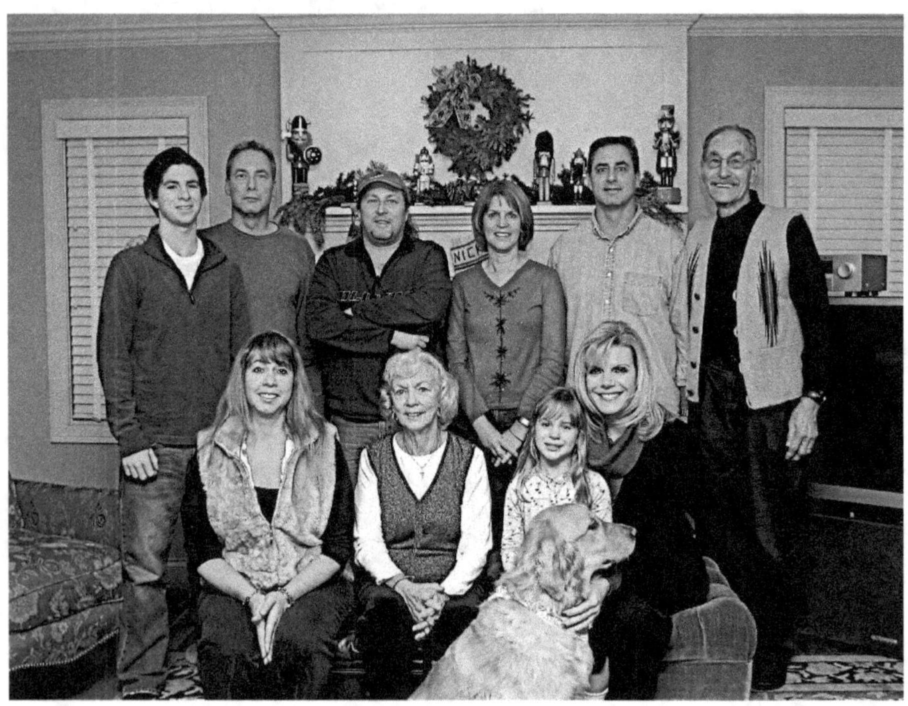

Familial love is inherent in family. Where there is love there is forgiveness and where there is forgiveness there is peace in the soul. The chain of generations is strong and impervious to separation. There is understanding of the value and importance of roots. The family transcends extinction.

— Thomas J. Rillo

About the Artist

Br. Martin Erspamer, OSB, is a monk of Saint Meinrad Archabbey in Saint Meinrad, Indiana. He is a highly respected and well-known liturgical artist who finds God in his artist studio. Br. Martin was formerly a Marianist Brother who worked in the Marianist Art Studio in St. Louis, Missouri. He has been a monk of Saint Meinrad for over 12 years. He was introduced to Saint Meinrad in 1996 during the Archabbey Church renovation. His expertise with stained glass windows was utilized during the renovation. He then made his canonical transfer to Saint Meinrad Archabbey. He works in a variety of media including stained glass windows, ceramics, prints, drawing, furniture, and pottery. He continues to work as a designer and painter of glass for Emil Frei in a stained glass studio located in St. Louis.

Br. Martin has always been very supportive of the Benedictine Oblate Community of Saint Meinrad Archabbey, and he has illustrated this book because of his interest and friendship with the author. The book, *The Work of Our hands: The Art of Martin Erspamer* is a wonderful testimony to his creative liturgical art.

The illustrations presented in this book are deeply appreciated and sincere gratitude is extended to Br. Martin Erspamer, OSB, for the generous contribution of his artwork.

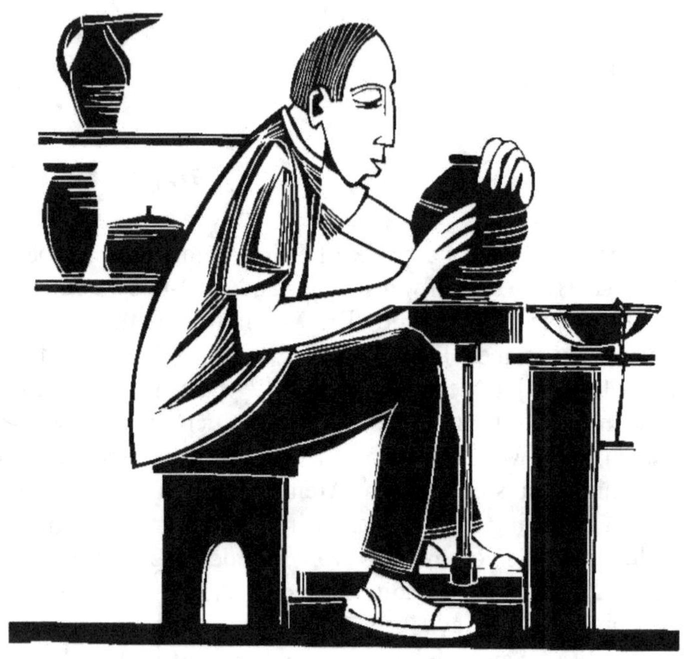

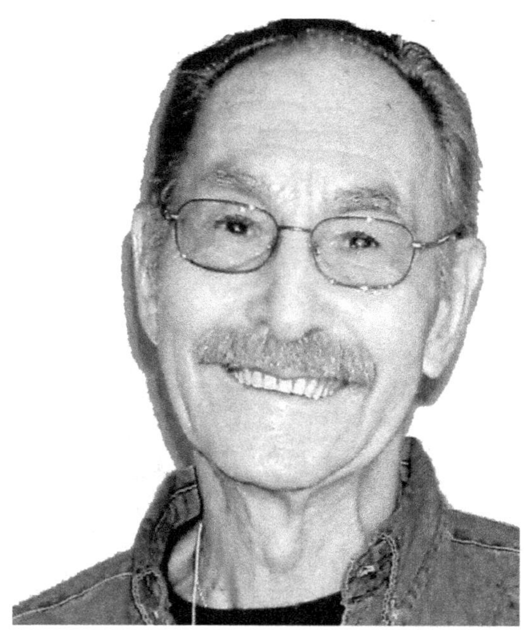

About the Author

The author is a retired professor from Indiana University. He was an environmental education professor for over 46 years. The author began writing this book when his wife Joan was diagnosed an Alzheimer's patient. Their lives changed dramatically. From vibrant active lives to lives that were limited in travel and social activities. The author first cared for his wife at home for a period of 4 years. This was total caregiving and he did everything that was required of care for Joan and maintenance of the home. Joan had two serious falls and it was recommended by the primary doctor and family members that she be admitted to an Alzheimer's Care Facility for the safety and protection of both caregiver and AD patient. It was at the time of Joan's admittance to the facility that the author felt the call to write about his experiences with caring for someone with AD. There are hardly any books written by someone who has coped with the challenges of care with AD as a focus.

The author was certified as a personal trainer in rehabilitative exercises for individuals with disorders of the brain. This background served him well in his research of AD. He learned a great deal from the many resources he utilized. Also, spending many hours living for six or seven hours in the Alzheimer's care unit, the author observed first-hand the progression of AD. This first-hand empirical research proved to be invaluable.

It is anticipated that the contents of this little book will be of help to caregivers who are coping, as the author did, with spousal care of AD patients.

Also from this author:

Deepening Faith Through Poetry (2008)

Thoughts for the Listening Heart (2011)

Growing Closer to God Through Poetry (2012)

Harden Not Your Hearts (2014)

Lift Up Your Hearts (2014)

Surrender in Trust (2015)

An Oblate's Commentaries on Benedictine Spirituality (2015)

A Knapsack of Poems for Lovers of the Outdoors (2016)

God Calls Us: A Collection of Prayers as Poems (2016)

Not Finished Just Begun: Recollections of a Life (2016)

God Is My Lifeline (2017)

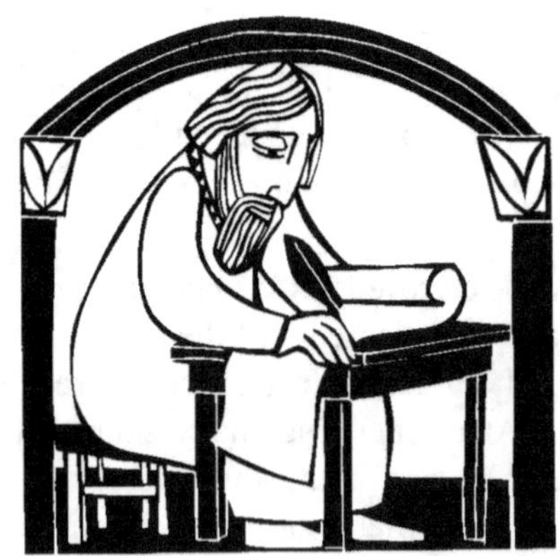

On the back cover: photo by Bill Bennett, now Director of IU Alumni Travel.